RECLAIMING
Vitality

A HEALING JOURNEY THROUGH
CHRONIC FATIGUE AND BURNOUT

SAMANTHA KEEN, M.A.

Copyright © 2024 by Samantha Keen.
All rights reserved. This book or any portion thereof may not be reproduced or used in any manner whatsoever without the express written permission of the publisher except for the use of brief quotations in a book review.

Publishing Services provided by Paper Raven Books LLC
Printed in the United States of America
First Printing, 2024

ISBN 979-8-9911119-0-4
Cover image by Yohanna Jessup

CONTENTS

Introduction 1

Chapter 1: In the Beginning, My Story 17

Chapter 2: Discover Subtle Bodies and Awakening 37

Chapter 3: Adventures of Consciousness and the Metaphysical Dimension of Healing 45

Chapter 4: Discovering the Crash & the Road to Recovery 61

Chapter 5: Centers of Energy Above the Head and CFS 77

Chapter 6: Yinyang Flow States and Recovery 95

Chapter 7: Technology &the Modern Age Contributing to the Fatigue Epidemic 131

Chapter 8: Harnessing the Powerof Noble Chaos (and Sleep) .. 157

Chapter 9: What Can You Do to Recover the Refreshing Power of Sleep? 185

Chapter 10: Willpower and Recovering a Healthy Creative Flow 209

Chapter 11: The Power of Truth 231

Addendum: With a Little Help From My Friends 246

A Glimpse of What Comes Next: Free Resources 249

Bibliography 251

Acknowledgements 261

INTRODUCTION

Remember when you used to wake up in the morning and roll out of bed happy to approach the day? And you felt full of life force, refreshed, and even joyful?

Now maybe you are exhausted, and you have been for a long time. Sleeping and resting do not seem to help. Or you do get better at times after a lot of rest, but then you crash again. In fact the crashing has become something of a lifestyle, and you really don't know how that happened. You were alive, you felt energized and vital, and then you got sick, and never really recovered even though the doctors and medical professionals couldn't find a true cause of the problem.

Perhaps when you try to restart your exercise program, you end up bedridden for days, or at least get markedly sicker for a time, even though earlier in your life exercise really wasn't a problem. Some of you may have even been very sporty, but now a fraction of that exercise sends your body reeling.

And for some of you, the brain fog might make you think that perhaps you are having some kind of midlife short-term memory issues. It is like a hangover that doesn't seem to lift with coffee at all, as it used to. In fact the coffee now makes you sick, just like so many other of your favorite foods, drinks, and substances.

Many of you will have seen alternative medical professionals, healers, and even therapists, sometimes paying ridiculous amounts of money just because you are so desperate to get better. These treatments may have helped the symptoms, to a degree. But treating the symptoms never really cured the underlying issue. And the underlying issue is still a mystery.

You may in fact be deeply frustrated, like I and many of the clients that I have seen were too. Angry that you feel chronically drained and that something as simple as a Zoom meeting or a trip to the mall can leave you laid out in bed or severely hindered for days.

The attempt to recover can also end up like a huge punishment, removing any possible triggers from your lifestyle until you eventually feel very alone and perhaps even more exhausted.

You might be like some of the young people I have known who had hours of morning routines daily because they were taking so many supplements, shakes, and treatments. If you are like that, you might also find yourself having to drag around huge bags of supplements and special foods anytime you need to travel.

Here you will not have to drag around bags of supplements and special foods, and if you are already doing that, then this is totally fine and not in conflict. What I want to share with you here is not a replacement for all the other treatments that you might try or have already tried. It's something that works on a different level than what you have been doing so far.

Perhaps you have been diagnosed with Chronic Fatigue Syndrome (CFS) or Myalgic Encephalomyelitis (ME), as I was. Or you are experiencing severe burnout or Long COVID or another form of post-viral fatigue. And you are in severe pain, collapsing regularly but finding ways to cope so that you don't have to let anyone but those closest to you know what is going on.

The word "crash" and the experience of an energetic collapse of some kind resonated with the direct experience of many of the hundreds of people that I have worked with and interviewed over the past 20 years about severe fatigue, including CFS and burnout.

When I started my studies in this area in 2003, the words *crash* and *collapse* were not used about these illnesses, but now the CDC uses them to describe what is called post-exertional malaise (PEM):

What is Post-Exertional Malaise (PEM)?

PEM is worsening of ME/CFS symptoms after physical or mental activity that wouldn't have caused problems previously. During PEM, ME/CFS symptoms may get worse or appear for the first time.

Symptoms may include:

- *Difficulty thinking*
- *Problems sleeping*
- *Headaches*
- *Feeling dizzy*
- *Severe tiredness*

It may take days, weeks, or longer to recover from PEM. People with ME/CFS often describe this experience as a "crash," "relapse," or "collapse."[1]

---

1. "Fast Facts: ME/CFS," Centers for Disease Control and Prevention, May 30, 2024, https://www.cdc.gov/me-cfs/about/fast-facts-about-me-cfs.html.

In the following chapters, I will describe what it means to crash or collapse from a unique perspective. It will illuminate some key pieces of the experience that will both allow you to recover a lot more quickly and also learn to sidestep the crashing altogether.

This is a proposal that the exploration of energetic and subtle aspects of the human body can help some people to recover from these illnesses. It is not meant to replace a physical diagnosis, nor the accompanying treatments. This is an additional lens through which to see the illness and the fatigue and in some cases find a pathway to full recovery.

More than anything, I feel that we are in a time when it is imperative to understand a holistic approach to illness.

If you have fully explored a Western approach to your fatigue, and it is not working, it is possible that seeing the issue through an understanding of the energetic or subtle aspects of your system could really help you to recover. This is an invitation to explore, to ask questions, and to see through the lens of a few different models. By all means take what is useful for you and apply it, and throw the rest away.

In all of the exploration and discovery along my own path, there was one thread that led me forward in the healing process, which was understanding the subtle-body mechanisms behind these little-understood conditions. "Subtle bodies" is a term used by Samuel Sagan, MD, (founder of the Clairvision School of Meditation) in his online correspondence course *KT Subtle Bodies, the Fourfold Model,* and it is this model I will use to talk about subtle bodies.

This model of subtle bodies describes the nonphysical aspects of human anatomy and physiology drawing from Western and Eastern models of subtle energy.

A key concept here is that the energy of life is one big part of the missing link in our understanding of fatigue and so many conditions that come out of it. The other part of the missing link is understanding consciousness, not just as psychology or thoughts and emotions, but also as energy that interacts with our vitality or life force at a very deep level.

Understanding subtle bodies shows us that the relationship between the energetic component of vitality and consciousness is fundamental to human existence but also all sorts of health-related dysfunctions: fatigue, the ability to recover quickly from illnesses and physical injuries, the ability to let go, much of the sexual dysfunction that people experience in the modern day, many unexplained digestion issues, and the inability to sit still and truly connect with ourselves.

The term subtle bodies as it is used in this book refers to, "The nonphysical layers which, together with the physical body, constitute a human being. Subtle bodies form the nonphysical hardware of consciousness."[2]

---

2. Samuel Sagan, *A Language to Map Consciousness*, Clairvision School, accessed June 11, 2024, https://clairvision.org/books/altmc/a-language-to-map-consciousness.html.

You might be skeptical about the existence of subtle energies and subtle bodies, as I was too. But this all changed when I had some profound experiences that opened up my own perception of how the crashing and collapsing was working in my body. In my search for recovery, I realized that I was missing a key piece of knowledge that many people in the world today are also in the dark about.

For myself this missing link first became clear when I had a kind of awakening in the year 2000, after nearly three years of debilitating fatigue, brain fog, post-exertion malaise (PEM), majorly uncomfortable digestive issues, and migraines, among other things. I had traveled the world and seen many doctors and alternative health professionals to find answers about what was happening, but at that point I still did not yet have a proper diagnosis.

That weekend I was meditating at a silent retreat just outside of London, UK, and I came down with one of the obliterating headaches that I had been suffering from since the onset of "whatever it was that had been happening to me" for the previous few years.

As I was in a meditation retreat, I was in complete silence. In the silence, I watched the excruciating pain come on. I noticed that while I was sitting, just observing my breath in stillness, that something inside me seemed to collapse.

I had no knowledge at that time of anything to do with "energy or qi or prana." I was a financial journalist with a scientist for a mother and a businessman for a father. For me "energy or qi" seemed vague at best and probably just a bit too "woo woo" for any serious consideration.

Nevertheless, I had a light bulb moment, sitting in total stillness and silence, watching the breath move in and out of my nose, seeing the pain slowly (but not so slowly, really, as it happened through the course of one day) descend into my body until I felt crippled. This was what my teacher in holistic counseling in Sydney, Australia later called an "aha moment." It was a deep realization that this problem that I was suffering from was not emotional or physical; it was energetic. This was a knowing that felt like a click inside of me.

After that day, I knew I had to learn about "energy," although I still did not know what that really meant. And I had to find out if there was a pathway to recover through understanding my own energy or what some people know as life force, "qi," and others as "prana."

Understanding subtle energetic mechanisms and how I could heal and cultivate my own life force was absolutely key in the journey of fully recovering from CFS, even after a diagnosis which essentially amounted to a doctor telling me that, "You have Chronic Fatigue Syndrome, and you will have to learn to live with it."

Defying that diagnosis, I went on to fully recover and then study the energetic and spiritual side of the suite of fatigue-related illnesses, such as CFS/ME, burnout, and other chronic unexplained conditions roughly under the same umbrella. I toured the world, gave talks and workshops, and worked with hundreds of people in one-on-one sessions as a practitioner in Inner Space Techniques (IST) and an instructor of the Clairvision School of Meditation.

In the 20 years of research that I have conducted on CFS, I also came across many people with burnout and even post-viral fatigue, and more recently Long COVID, that fit into a similar energetic category as the people who with CFS who were finding recovery from working underlying energetic issues that contributed to their illness in the first place.

I came to see these illnesses as a loosely grouped set of diagnoses that have some energetic crossover, much like a Venn diagram. In the crossover where these illnesses meet in this vision, some people with one or more of these diagnoses can have significant recovery through exploring and treating the subtle bodies or energetic level of the condition.

My point here is that knowledge of the subtle body and energetic component of these categories of illness is an additional tool that really worked for me, and for many others that I have either witnessed or worked with myself as an IST practitioner. While modern Western medicine is important and a marvel in many cases, it does not yet know how to treat every condition successfully, and in the case of these particular illnesses doesn't pinpoint what the real cause of the problem is. In this case, I would like to put forward that it is worth considering exploring the condition from this bigger perspective of the human body.

To help you understand what I mean here, I have written this book using my own experiences of CFS and Long COVID, as well the case studies of many others, some of them diagnosed with burnout or post-viral fatigue. In all cases people were consulting their doctors and using Western medicine as much as possible to treat their condition. Many times, including for myself, this did not lead them to the road of recovery, and so we tried different approaches in the attempt to get better.

As part of this energetic approach, a fundamental aspect of my recovery and many others that I have worked together with over the years has been the foundational technique of uplifting, or pulling up heavy, dark fatigue out of the body of life or vitality. This is a technique that addresses fatigue which is not just your standard physical tiredness at the end of the day. It is a fatigue that results more from the ongoing gripping and tension of the unconscious intensity that many people with CFS are dealing with. They don't have a language for it, or a clear sense of how to address it. But when you talk to many people with CFS types of illnesses, they absolutely get the idea that their own intensity is crashing into them and causing these incredibly difficult symptoms.

Finding uplifting and applying it has been so foundational in my own recovery and that of many others I have interviewed or worked with as a private IST practitioner that I really am so happy to introduce this concept for you here in this book, including the whole context of understanding subtle bodies that goes with the technique. This technique can be applied even for those who are very unwell and bedridden in the earlier or more severe phases of the illness.

As CFS and burnout often have multiple layers of cause, there can be more than one way to treat such a condition. In my own recovery there were several different stages of return to full health and vitality.

After the initial very severe phase of being bedridden, a major part of my own journey and that of many others I've worked with or interviewed was learning how to connect deeply with the principle of life by fully letting go.

I bet you can relate to the fact that stress, tension, and gripping create or exacerbate illness. For those with CFS and some types of burnout or Long COVID, this incredible tension sometimes creates such severe symptoms that it can even be life-threatening when at its worst.

Even though grasping tension in the mind and the body is a central mechanism of consciousness in modern life, I bet you have also experienced the relief that comes with letting go of all that physical and emotional stress. In over two decades of exploration, I learned that we all share the primal desire to let go, to spread, to merge, to feel that blissful feeling when you just allow your consciousness to dive into nature or another person and become one in such a way that you feel a total release.

This is the desire for sex, for a good night of sleep, for a great vacation on an island somewhere, or for the deep dive into nature that takes you away from the stress of everything in your life. For others, it takes the form of a deep inner realization of Peace, a spiritual experience that releases them from suffering.

This merging into a blissful state is one way that we can be deeply refreshed, rejuvenated, and renewed. Yet people are increasingly finding it hard to have this kind of reset.

What I have found working with thousands of people around the world is that we get stuck in "grasping," tension, gripping, or some kind of contraction. Most of us at one time or another have experienced a phase when we cannot help but hold on. And so when we do try to sleep, even if it is for hours or even days at a time, we are not able to experience refreshment or rejuvenation.

In the (not so) distant past, this letting go into the essence of aliveness that is really inside all of us happened unconsciously. But as we move further and further into the technological age, we need to learn to let go consciously, to choose letting go.

Rediscovering the profound and yet simple joy of truly releasing all that unconscious tension and stress is one of the fundamental things that I want to share with you in the journey of this book. Letting go means learning to consciously allow ourselves to go into a primordial chaos. This is like a kind of churning of the body of energy that affords a huge state of regeneration.

That is why I am proposing that this is a Noble Cure, a pathway to understanding subtle energies, including the primordial beauty of our own body of life force, how it interacts with the grasping mind and the relief and deep peace we experience when we can consciously choose to just let go. In understanding those levels of our own subtle energies, we can then learn how to cultivate this precious essence of life inside of us, and the deep calm that it can bring.

The next step in the recovery process is that of developing the ability to get things done with a connected sense of flow, meaning that the doing does not reignite this massive tension inside that creates the sickness and the crashing of vitality.

The Chinese model of yinyang[3] flow, both the opposition and the complementarity, is so helpful here. In this yinyang model, we're all feminine and masculine all of the time, but at any one moment we tend towards one or the other polarity.

These forces within us are also outside of us. And if we push against this flow, then it can enhance the tension or friction that tends towards creating the crash symptoms. So we need to learn to flow with the forces of masculine and feminine inside of us, sometimes needing to be driven and pointed, sometimes more receptive and peripheral, resting and letting go.

---

3. From Robin R. Wang's usage of the term. Wang uses the term "yinyang," rather than "yin or yang," "yin-yang," or "yin and yang." This reflects the Chinese usage, in which the terms are directly set together and would not be linked by a conjunction.

In this flow, the power of knowing what you want or desire is key because when you do what you really want—not the surface or externally conditioned desires that leave you empty and deflated, but the true wantings that come from deep inside—then you have more energy. People get things done when they are connected to the energy of wantings and desires. When you really want something, you find the energy to achieve it. This is a simple and yet powerful way to move forward with recovery, once you have the techniques of energy management under your belt.

The last chapter explores the power of truth in finding the way to recovery. This is a simple and beautiful teaching that can help many people find their way to shifting their relationship to CFS and burnout. For me, it was really instrumental in finding the steps to recovery.

Before I got sick with CFS, I had no thought nor even any idea of a spiritual path, let alone meditation. And when I got sick, I would never have dreamed that these things would lead me to a full recovery from the same unbearable illness.

Not just any old meditation and spiritual path, but a path that showed me how to heal the condition at the level of my own energy or life force. Finding meditation and spirituality was profound, but it was also practical. This was a path that unfolded in a series of steps that resulted in my recovery and so much more.

Since then, I have discovered that many people find wellness and freedom through spiritual work and meditation in a very real way. I saw this shared experience through interviewing more than 100 people about their experiences with CFS and burnout, as well as completing thousands of private sessions with people around the world, working as an IST practitioner for more than 20 years.

Lisa Miller, PhD, in her book *The Awakened Brain: The New Science of Spirituality and our Quest for an Inspired Life*, says that her breakthrough MRI findings showed that each of us has what she calls an 'awakened brain.'

Each of us is endowed with the natural capacity to perceive a greater reality and consciously connect to the life force that moves in, through, and around us. Whether or not we participate in a spiritual practice or adhere to a faith tradition, whether or not we identify as religious or spiritual, our brain has a natural inclination toward and docking station for spiritual awareness.[4]

Miller describes the awakened brain as the "neutral circuitry that allows us to see the world more fully and thus enhance our individual, societal and global wellbeing."[5]

In this book, Miller also says, "I've discovered that the awakened brain is both inherent to our physiology and invaluable to our health and functioning."[6]

---

4. Lisa Miller PhD, *The Awakened Brain: The New Science of Spirituality and Our Quest for an Inspired Life* (New York: Random House, 2021), 7.
5. Lisa Miller, *The Awakened Brain*, 8.
6. Lisa Miller, *The Awakened Brain*, 9.

When I read about this, I was fascinated because Miller carefully lays out what I already knew to be true from years on the ground facilitating people to find and explore this in themselves.

Let me start at the beginning...

1

IN THE BEGINNING, MY STORY

Perhaps like me, you have a pattern of fighting to the top, chasing that euphoric high, until you crash and seriously burn out, taking what seems like an unusually long time to recover.

For me, full recovery from this pattern would only come through a complete shift inside of myself, when I started to understand my own subtle energies, and my relationship with my own willpower.

In that awakening, and the healing of my body, my experience of the world would be filled out like a picture postcard becoming a full 3D virtual image, bursting with the vibrancy of life. I came through that dark night of the soul to learn about my own spirituality and how it could be cultivated actively through engaging my subtle energy bodies using meditation techniques.

When I first had the impulse to write this book and do this work, the main thing that I wanted to share was that you can recover from the debilitating and bone-aching exhaustion of Chronic Fatigue Syndrome or Myalgic Encephalomyelitis (CFS/ME).

Whether you believe it or not right now, I want you to know that yes, you can get better, be more alive, have more energy, and experience hope and enthusiasm again in your life!

This epiphany first popped into my head when I really knew I was fully recovered from CFS. In that moment, there were clear vast blue skies above and all around me, as I drove across the rich red Australian desert. I was driving 12 hours to Sydney from White Cliffs in New South Wales, where I had been studying meditation and transformation full-time for 18 months at a retreat center directly with Dr. Samuel Sagan. I felt absolutely free, liberated of the pain and heavy brain fog, as well as numerous other symptoms that had plagued me during the previous five years of struggle with CFS.

Freedom after all that pain and suffering was so liberating that I decided then I wanted to share it with others who were feeling hopeless, hitting walls with burnout and ongoing, unexplained debilitating fatigue. I was feeling completely alive, and full of vitality, recovered from years of sleep issues, exhaustion, being plagued with overwhelming sensitivities and allergies, migraines, brain fog, and bouts of flu-like symptoms.

Since my own recovery, I have lived in five different cities, in four different countries, on three different continents. I became an IST practitioner and taught many workshops in meditation around the world, seeing thousands of private clients from all walks of life, and wrote a master's thesis on the topic of recovering from CFS using the understanding of subtle bodies. Not to mention immigrating from Australia to the USA and falling in love a few times along the way.

Sharing my story of illness and recovery from chronic fatigue with you is intended to inspire you in case you are exhausted, drained, and feeling hopeless about your own path.

If you are burnt out, struggling with brain fog, dragging your body around with little sign of relief, or crashing on a regular basis in such a way that you end up in bed for long stretches not really knowing why, then this story is intended to convey a sense of possibility and victory.

It is important because now debilitating fatigue including CFS/ME, Long COVID and chronic situations of burnout have reached epidemic proportions around the world.

BEFORE I WAS SICK

Spinning back even earlier to 1995, before I was really sick, I was 23 years old, feeling a different kind of freedom, on a three-day journey across Australia, through that blistering red desert, this time on a bus from Perth in Western Australia, to Sydney in New South Wales on the other side of the country. I left my childhood home to go to the biggest city in Australia at the time, where I knew nobody. I was en-route to not only the career that I thought I wanted, but also a huge crash and then a spiritual awakening that would change everything.

That three-day journey across the desert felt like a transition through fire. By the time I arrived at my destination, the whites of my eyes had turned completely red, bloodshot from the brutal intensity of the bus air-conditioning. I guessed that desert temperatures over 105 F meant that they had some kind of refrigeration system blowing that dry air at us to keep us alive on the journey.

At that time I had no concept of anything spiritual or energetic at all. Instead I was en-route to an outer kind of success, one that came at a price.

On that bus, I was not sick, but I was on my way towards it. The stubborn will, the desperate desire to prove my worth, the wide-eyed enthusiasm about the world would lead me to fight harder than my body could possibly handle.

The pushing and the drive that got me onto that bus and that would eventually get me into the career as a journalist were definitely instrumental to the unexplained devastating levels of fatigue and physical pain that were to come.

I was living in one of the most magnificent cities in the world, desperately wanting to be great at a time when it was becoming increasingly difficult to get into print media without contacts and inroads. Print media was dying, and the internet was being birthed.

Just under a year after my arrival, I became a financial journalist working for an accounting newspaper, and within two years, I was working in the fast-paced wire industry getting news out second by second, living the dream.

That lifestyle of striving for the top and winning was so fun for me at the time. While my articles were published daily in newspapers around the country, I lived in an apartment near Bronte Beach where I went bodysurfing in the mornings and then caught the bus into the hectic high-rise building. I would arrive early in the office to read the three or four (physical) newspapers, while drinking my coffee and eating my huge chunks of sourdough toast. Yes physical newspapers, coffee, and buttered toast with Vegemite. (Side note: it has been a long time since I had any of those things!)

It was the beginning of the internet, the dawn of the new wave of media, and everything was happening at once. There were three computers on my desk, two phones, and a lot of manic noise in the newsroom as everyone was working at breakneck speed to get the stories out faster than humanly possible while also being more accurate than any of our competitors.

It was so competitive that I used to describe a press pack interviewing one person for the same story as akin to a group of football players dressed in jackets and nice shoes. Nothing like running from a conference or an AGM (Annual General Meeting) at breakneck speed to call in a story to the editor while the competitors all did the same in the other corners of the room. Definitely an adrenaline buzz.

Then I crashed!

THE CRASH OF A SHOOTING STAR— OR SO I BELIEVED

Starting to get the picture of an adrenaline junkie yet? Perhaps you have your own version of this story?

But then after three years in that industry, just when I was becoming a shooting star, within reach of fame and recognition, I crashed, and I crashed hard. I got really sick, and it went on for a long time. I was dragging my body to and from work, falling asleep at the desk, pulled by a deep, heavy, foggy fatigue that did not leave me for several years. There were digestive issues that were painful, aggressive, embarrassing, and uncomfortable. Headaches of far greater severity than I had ever had before, unexplained fevers, aches, and pains. Most of all the strange situation that, for the first time in my very active life, exercise made me much worse, not better.

I later found out that this crash was more than just a physical virus at the time. I probably had Epstein-Barr as years later this came up in tests. But even when I did everything to address that illness—cleansing, diets, detox, resting, changing my lifestyle—I did not get better. There was an energetic component that turned out to be key to my return to wellbeing.

For the first couple of years of the illness, I fought hard to find a diagnosis and cure, trying everything from specialists in Sydney, Australia, and London, UK to many different types of alternative doctors and healers. I moved countries—I was a fighter after all. This was how I generally rolled in my life. I changed jobs, I took time off, I rested, and I stopped eating any foods that seemed to make my symptoms worse. At times the so-called food intolerance issues resulted in a very basic diet of brown rice and selected steamed vegetables.

That little bit of relief that came out of so much focus on my health wasn't enough for me. I wanted a full recovery. I was adamant that it was possible because I had been physically fit and healthy before, and then for no apparent reason, I was debilitated, clouded in a heavy sleepy fog, plagued with constant headaches, drained by food and chemical sensitivities beyond what I had thought possible, and my bowels seemed to be incapable of doing much more than embarrassing me in every way possible.

I would not give up until I was fully recovered. What I did not know, though, was that by the time I was recovered, I would be a completely different person, and yet so much more myself.

EVERYTHING BEGAN TO CHANGE

A huge part of my own recovery was finding a spiritual path of real substance.

Central to the theory that human beings have subtle bodies, or nonphysical aspects to their existence, is the experience of ourselves as spiritual beings. The age-old dilemma of being both an animal and an angel in one body has been the motivator for many mythologies and religions across the ages and throughout different cultures around the world.

When I was still struggling with CFS, and had no real belief in anything spiritual or religious at all, I had a kind of awakening in June 1999. I returned to the place of my birth: Malawi, Africa. After several years of illness, being in bed a lot, and in pain even more, I just decided to do something I had really wanted to do for many years. I went on an epic journey to the place where I'd spent the first few years of my life, returning for the first time since my family left to immigrate to Australia in 1976. That was when my recovery really began.

I had been sick for several years, searched for answers in Australia and the UK, and finally just went on a backpacking trip regardless of the symptoms that plagued me. A couple of doctors thought I was mad. And maybe from a rational standpoint, I was. But sometimes you have to do what you have to do.

After a month of journeying through Zimbabwe and Zambia, I was in Malawi, when I had a really big shift of consciousness. What should have been a three-hour journey took me and two completely new backpacking friends more than 14 hours. A bus that had been very difficult to find in the first place that was supposed to take us to the lake just stopped halfway there in the middle of nowhere and dumped us and all the passengers on the side of the road. For the local people, I did not get the sense this was out of the ordinary. But for myself and my two young English companions at the time, this was really outside of our comfort zone.

We ended up backpacking, busing, hitchhiking and even walking to find our way from Lilongwe to a small village on the edge of Lake Malawi, one of the biggest freshwater lakes in the world. When we finally made it to the lake, we were sitting on the back of an open truck holding on fiercely for our lives as it bounced through the outback dirt road. The sun was setting on one side of the truck and the moon rising on the other.

I remembered a poem or prayer by Michael Leunig, the Australian cartoonist and philosopher:

> *There are only two feelings*
> *Love and fear.*
> *There are only two languages,*
> *Love and fear.*
> *There are only two activities,*
> *Love and fear.*
> *There are only two motives,*
> *two procedures, two frameworks,*
> *two results.*
> *Love and fear.*
> *Love and fear.*[7]

Symbolically, on one side of the truck, there sat the golden flames of the sun looming brilliant over the Malawi landscape and on the other side of us the moon, its full silvery white sister, rising over the lake. The lake I had heard about my whole life, so big it looks like an ocean. I was awake to the choice in myself to see things one way or another, either full of love or brimming with fear.

There were no phones, no banks, no way to get money, no way to contact anyone, and I was here with two complete strangers who were now my brothers. I had never felt so alive in my life. I chose love.

A few days later, when I danced on a tiny island in the middle of Lake Malawi as the soft pitter-patter of summer

---

7. Michael Leunig, "Prayers," Leunig, accessed June 11, 2024, https://www.leunig.com.au/works/prayers.

rain hit the grass roof of our open-air shelter, I felt like I was dancing in the sky with the sea eagles that swooped in around us for the fish fed to them by the two men who had rowed me across the lake. In that moment, truly alone, and truly connected, there was only joy and physically a sense of no limits, and there was no CFS. I was awake to myself in a way that I had never been before. It was the beginning of a new phase, a discovery of my inner self as a pathway to the fullness of life and light.

Somewhere in the following two weeks between Lake Malawi, meeting another old friend and my original traveling companion at a hostel in Blantyre, and then traveling together on a bus through Mozambique, seeing children eat roasted rats on a skewer, and arriving back in Zimbabwe, I realized that I had changed. I was a different person. It was not just a profound memory; it was an experience that had enlarged me and given me more breadth of being.

When I returned to London, I remained symptom-free for a month or so, and then the crashing returned. This time, they were not constant heavy dark crashes that went on for months, but still days or weeks of pain and suffering that just happened as part of my ongoing experience of life. I was shifting in and out of wellness and illness pretty quickly and unexpectedly.

The inner shift that happened in Africa had brought with it the realization that I had to meditate. It is hard to explain because it was not a rational idea, but more on the silent level of a flash of intuition.

Something inside me had cracked open when I went to Africa and traveled around, meeting people and seeing how they lived. I realized firstly how small my problems were. Really so small and the solutions seemed very possible. I no longer felt defeated by the illness. My Spirit soared with enthusiasm and the need to just become that different person that I had felt in Malawi, the person with no limits.

Looking back, it is clear that through those years when I was really sick, the CFS seemed to lift off of me completely for days and even weeks sometimes when I traveled to places of great natural beauty and when I exceeded my own expectations of what was possible for me.

In the model of subtle bodies that I will unpack more as we go, that liftoff of the CFS symptoms, so to speak, was because I was immersed in natural environments full of life force. I was in spectacular landscapes like the Alps, or the Zambezi River, or Victoria Falls. These are places where the power of life is so immense it would boost my energy and life force in a very positive way.

When I returned to London after the trip to Malawi, I proceeded to change around my whole life so that I could meditate. That meant switching to a part-time job editing a finance magazine, leaving my husband at the time, and joining a group called Friends of the Western Buddhist Order

(FWBO), attending classes several times a week as well as going to silent meditation retreats whenever possible.

In that year after the trip to east Africa, working in London, meditating and going to yoga classes, life took on a newfound simplicity. It was a massive relief. I could feel myself get tangibly lighter. My yoga postures became easier; my diet became simpler. There was a joy in the whole thing that lifted me up. And there were new friends who were also passionate about meditation and transformation. They were all battling with their own demons and sincerely wanting to grow and open their hearts. I loved them; they loved me. The world opened up to be a friendlier and warmer place.

There were still times, though, when I got sick, I crashed, and the pain and misery came back.

None of this was consciously about getting better from the illness; it was just taking steps towards something that I wanted that was coming from the inside of me, not an external expectation that I was trying to shape myself towards.

Meditation was like a switch that went on inside of me and never turned off again.

A NEWFOUND PASSION FOR MEDITATION – AND RECOVERY!

Finding meditation was the beginning of my journey to full recovery.

I am not alone in finding recovery as part of a bigger spiritual awakening. Psychologist Lisa Miller documents scientific studies that show we are biologically hardwired for spiritual connection.

> *Spirituality is an inner sense of relationship to a higher power that is loving and guiding. The word we give to this higher power might be God, nature, spirit, the universe, the creator, or other words that represent a divine presence. But the important point is that spirituality encompasses our relationship and dialogue with this higher presence.*[8]

This journey inside of myself, a spiritual awakening that was to continue for the rest of my life, started to give me a sense of how to move towards full recovery. I was immediately passionate about meditation, not because I thought it would make me better but because the immense frustration of my health journey had somehow led me to this totally different place in my life where going inside and

---

8. Lisa Miller and Teresa Barker, *The Spiritual Child: The New Science on Parenting for Health and Lifelong Thriving* (New York: Picador/St. Martin's Press, 2016), 25.

finding real peace was the only thing that seemed to make sense. Along the way, I also saw a lot about what was blocking that inner peace.

One weekend on a silent retreat with a group of Buddhist meditators, I had another big insight or flash of intuition that opened up the recovery process at another level.

It was two days of silence, watching the breath move in and out, sitting in a little old house, a bus ride from my flat in East London. Feeling awkward, I sat with about 15 others as I tried to follow the instructions of a senior Buddhist man and woman.

I was really new to all of this. Listening to the soft hum of my breath, trying to silence the mind, noticing every single thought and tension as it moved in and out of my awareness. It had begun to dawn on me that my internal space of consciousness was so rich and at times even tempestuous. But more than that, my mind was also sometimes really bloody loud!

About halfway in, earnestly sitting still, I started to feel like I was becoming heavier and heavier. Literally, it was as if I was watching the pain descend into me until I felt crushed. All through this, I also seemed to become more and more angry, frustrated, unhappy. I mean, I was in a lot of pain. And I do remember seeing the other silent retreat participants gently parting like waves to make space around me.

In other agonizing moments during that weekend, also sitting still, watching my breath move in and out of my body,

I was in total pain, and felt completely stuck. I was caught in emotions for long stretches, which felt like eons, but more likely were more like 15 or 20 minutes. And I was sick.

As I sat watching the breath, I just had this kind of epiphany. "This is energetic. It is not physical; it is not emotional." I did not have a context for energy at all. I knew nothing of life force, prana, or qi or nonphysical realities. But somehow my mind had opened enough, and perhaps in the Buddhist texts that I was reading, something was passing unconsciously. I just knew that my issue had to do with my energy.

That realization that my crash was energetic changed my life because it was a lead, something to find out more about, that would uncover the true cause of the CFS.

Yet at the same time, there were long moments of elevated inspiration full of depth and presence. The tranquility that filled the room seemed to be golden and complete rather than empty and scary. In the peace, it felt like there was a silent sound of internal singing, as if I was sitting in the quiet harmonies and high eloquent notes of angels.

I did not realize it, but I was starting to connect back with the silence and peace of my own higher self, the part of me that had been drowned out by my desperate grasping frustration to win. And it would be the key to many of my unanswered questions.

In the magnified awareness of meditation, I was seeing the experience of being in myself when I felt so healthy and well, contrasted with a crash or collapse into a state of grasping and pain. This disparity between the blissful states of wellbeing and peace with the intense grasping and pain fraught with frustration and other emotions and thoughts was a mirror of my whole life.

Seeing this apparent contradiction between the grasping pain and the deep inner wellbeing at more and more refined levels would be a very important key to my recovery. In that moment of epiphany about my energy, I was given the first clue to learning that I could change that pattern of swinging between wellness and extreme pain and illness. It was to take me to another style of meditation in Sydney where I would learn how to choose being grounded in myself more and more of the time until it became the norm.

It was completely unexpected that meditation helped me to find my way to recovery. When I started to meditate, it was a result of a desire to know myself and to learn to master stillness and peace. What I didn't expect was that while sitting there, through the ups and downs, I'd also begin to see things about the mysterious illness that had gripped me and find my way to techniques that would help me to recover.

It's easy to think that this crash might have an emotional cause, and there were certainly a number of people who suggested that it did. Before I had the diagnosis for CFS, there were people who tried to imply that the illness was a result of something emotional that I was doing to myself. To them it might have appeared like that because the illness came with an extra intensity of emotions, and so they thought my emotionality was the cause. But that was not right. In fact, it was narrow-minded, judgmental, and illustrated a lack of understanding of the illness and its cause.

However, there was something that they were (perhaps) trying to point to, which was that the road to recovery would require a lot of inner searching for me to really comprehend. I needed to have an open mind to see what was the real cause of this massive energetic collapse that had ruined my life at the time. What I found out was that it was energetic in its cause, not physical, and not emotional.

A SPIRITUAL COMPONENT TO MY RECOVERY

CFS is an umbrella term that covers numerous conditions and symptoms, and therefore there are a number of different ways that people recover from this illness.

The Centers for Disease Control and Prevention says:

ME/CFS is a biological illness that affects many body parts. It causes severe fatigue not improved by rest, problems thinking and sleeping, dizziness, pain, and many other symptoms. People with ME/CFS may not look sick but can't do their normal activities. ME/CFS may get worse after they do any activity—physical or mental. This symptom is called post-exertional malaise (PEM). After they exert themselves, they may need to stay in bed for an extended time. About 1 in 4 people with ME/CFS are confined to bed at some point in their illness.[9]

As far as the CDC was concerned at the time of writing, there was no cure or approved treatment for these conditions. However, the reality is that some people do get better and others do not.

In the 20 years that I have spent researching CFS, talking about it with groups and at workshops, interviewing and working as a practitioner with those who have this kind of illness, I saw a kind of crossover with a few other illnesses such as burnout, post-viral fatigue, and more recently Long COVID. Medical authorities and therapists of many kind had theories and treatments for these conditions yet in general have been mystified about what they really are and the real cause. I found that some of the people who fit into the umbrella of one or a few of these conditions did find recovery like me, through working on the subtle underlying energetic causes of their fatigue and other symptoms.

There are alternative therapists of all kinds who claim to have a cure, and they do work for some people. Many of us with these conditions try so many different things, and spend a lot of money on treatments that do not work before we find our way out. Some people do what my first doctor told me in

---

[9]. "ME/CFS Basics," Centers for Disease Control and Prevention, May 10, 2024, https://www.cdc.gov/me-cfs/about/index.html.

1997 when I went to complain of this mysterious condition, "learn to cope."

While I do see that the path to recovery all started for me with meditation, that is definitely not true for everyone who recovers.

However, the context of my recovery is important because when interviewing and then later working with people as a practitioner, I saw that many others with these illnesses have also found some kind of spiritual or meditative practice was important in their recovery.

2

DISCOVERING SUBTLE BODIES AND AWAKENING

Perhaps you already know firsthand that the first phases of illness with CFS or some very intense types of burnout are just so difficult. Maybe you have even experienced that kind of debilitating fatigue where just getting out of bed is near impossible?

Phase two of the illness is a little bit different because that is where you are up and down out of bed, some days better than others, some weeks in bed, some weeks able to semi-function in the world.

What I call phase two is where you might be more likely to start looking for alternative solutions to the health issue that plagues you. This is where I started to find meditation and knowledge of subtle bodies, and I was able to shift into recovery.

On the road to recovery, after finding meditation, I started to learn more about spirituality and energy, including concepts of qi, prana or life force. That is when I met Ruth-Helen Camden, IST practitioner, naturopath, and psychologist. Her brown curly hair was bouncing with the enthusiasm that shone out of her eyes as she shared about some of the things I was so fascinated to learn. She was teaching an introductory course in energetic healing at Nature Care College in Sydney, Australia.

I knew there was a missing piece to this puzzle, but I did not have the context to understand it at all. And then suddenly, that previously hidden context was being laid out in front of me in this course, piece by piece, giving the distinct sensation that a light bulb was turned on, illuminating a formerly dark room inside. It was a welcome blast of clarity after years of struggling in the fog of mysterious symptoms and unpredictable collapses.

That light bulb really came from Ruth-Helen, and her passion for Inner Space Techniques or IST, a modality of therapies based on meditation that brings a metaphysical dimension into a psychotherapeutic approach. Ruth-Helen had many modalities under her belt as a healer, but really favored IST because she found it worked at a deep level. Through her IST would become key to my journey of recovery, bringing a precision and clarity to my own ability to understand and rebuild my own subtle energetic vitality.

Later, I would become so passionate about this journey that I would go on to be an IST practitioner myself and help thousands of others on their own paths of healing and inner growth.

By the time I met Ruth-Helen, I had been through so much frustration and even depression about my symptoms that her positivity and bubbly encouragement was very welcome in my life.

Perhaps like you, I had fought for answers, given up, tried to accept the situation, and just plain settled for this angry painful existence. And now finally here was someone who had a model to describe what I called a crash. I am sure that you can imagine the relief I felt when she spoke to exactly what was happening inside me with such joyful confidence that I was completely lifted up out of my funk. It was a new birth of hope.

When I started to see Ruth-Helen for private sessions after the semester had completed, I realized that she expertly used IST with her one-on-one clients as a set of modalities to help people release stuck and blocked emotions, but also the energies behind those emotions.

I was so excited to hear that this system had a whole set of techniques developed just for people with CFS and burnout-type illnesses. A way to rebuild your energy and vitality. There is also a whole understanding within the model of how technology and modern-day issues like pollution and climate change impact our vital energy, and what to do about it.

There is a regression component to IST, but it is also backed by an in-depth model of subtle bodies or nonphysical aspects of the human body.

The fourfold model of subtle bodies used by Samuel Sagan, MD, is modeled on his own experiences and research with his students of Clairvision School. In addition to his own vision and experience, he drew from traditional Chinese medicine, Indian models of healing and meditation, and Western esoteric systems, deliberately using common terminology where possible to highlight similarities between different systems. Sagan's system also included a body of knowledge gained through direct experience of a group of meditators that included therapists, psychologists, business people, and others from diverse backgrounds.

The first time I went to see Ruth-Helen as a private client, I was simply curious about past-life regression, and while I did not necessarily believe in past lives at the time, I was open and wondering what it would be like.

Ruth-Helen, dressed in a chocolate-brown soft sweater and long flowing skirt, with bouncing soft brown curls, was bright, bubbly, and uplifting in her very presence. She made me laugh even as I described my misery. It was so invigorating to laugh at something that had weighed on me for years.

When she looked me deep in the eyes, she seemed to see right through my soul, cutting into the core of whatever I was saying like a knife through butter. I felt transparent, really understood, and embraced. It was easy to see how her clients would really like just being in her presence.

To begin, Ruth-Helen had me lay down on a mat, and she sat next to me on a cushion on the floor. She talked me through a series of steps into an experience of meditation. It was like being taken by the hand and led to a vast space inside of myself that was both familiar and unfamiliar. It had a feeling of softness and warmth.

She put her hand lightly on the center of my chest, the energetic heart center, and I went into the feelings there where I found sadness, loneliness, and an image of a little girl. The little girl was me, and Ruth-Helen encouraged me to feel into the child as me even though it wasn't anything that I had consciously remembered from this life. I spent some time feeling what the girl was feeling and sensing the whole experience. We went through the coldness of a cave, being abandoned by her family, and then the way that she died alone without ever knowing why they left her behind. I cried and cried.

It was such a deep felt sense of abandonment. The tears flowed for the whole session, and at the end there was a peaceful silence full of presence that felt so tender and filled up the darkness inside of me. It was all so beautiful and loving, and also very intense and painful.

After the years of meditation and CFS, it felt like a relief to let out all of that heavy emotion and feel the levity of the stillness at the end of the session. Then I went home and I cried more and more for the next few days until I returned to Ruth-Helen for the next visit. More tears and more tears were released. It took a couple more visits to get out the weight of this built-up emotion, but when it finally lifted, I felt washed and clean.

Later, when I spoke with Ruth-Helen about those first visits and the immense outpouring of grief that I went through after the sessions once I returned home, she told me that she was really surprised and impressed that I just allowed those emotions to flow, somehow understanding it was simply part of the process. I did not freak out that I was crying so much, because somewhere inside it was an immense relief to let go of that baggage. I understood that I had been carrying it around for a long time, and this was now the time to put it down, let it be washed away.

Many people with heavy fatigue and burnout have a lot of pent-up or repressed emotions from trauma in this life or past lives that has not been released. It was not just an emotional release, nor a physical shift. I was releasing blocked energy inside of me that had not moved in other styles of meditation.

Releasing that stuck energy with tears, anger, or whatever is needed to go deeper inside can be a tremendous relief, and even more than that, it can reveal a lot of vitality or life force. (From here when I talk about life or life force,

I am also referring to what is known as qi in the system of traditional Chinese medicine and prana in the Indian model.)

It certainly left me a lot lighter and wanting to release more and more of the unnecessary burdens inside. Things that were stuck in my life and seemed impossible began to move very fast after those first few sessions.

It didn't bother me that the techniques made me cry, that I felt sad, even heartbroken. Intuitively, I knew that this was what I needed to let go of that heavy baggage from the past, to release the blockages that kept pulling me back in the same way a rower might feel when trying to row a boat that remains anchored. It did not matter to me whether it was an actual past life or just something symbolic deep inside me that was coming up to the light of my own self-awareness to be released. My tears seemed to rinse away the dark weight that I was carrying in my heart.

Later, Ruth-Helen remarked to me that many people would not want to return for a second session after so much emotional outpouring. For me, though, after more than two years of intensive meditation including weeks at a time of silence, just feeling my stuff, I was so overwhelmingly grateful to have someone to help me with that stuff. It had been in my face while I sat through the silence, and I could not resolve it on my own. Now I had an expert who just helped me to let go. Wow, for me that was all I wanted to do.

3

ADVENTURES OF CONSCIOUSNESS, UNCHARTED TERRITORIES, AND THE METAPHYSICAL DIMENSION OF HEALING

A huge part of the second phase of CFS was about just finding that pathway to recover. And even more important in that phase was finding the pathway for releasing emotional and energetic blocks by diving into my own landscapes of consciousness using IST. This suite of techniques was the most exciting thing I had ever encountered because it facilitated a lightness of being that was so invigorating, I passionately wanted to share it with people like yourself.

In my own journey of recovery, the dropping of emotional baggage and healing of old wounds was instrumental to my recovery from CFS. Part of that journey was also discovering things about myself of which I had no inkling, including powerful, interesting, and mystical aspects of my inner self.

Weekly classes in Sydney were an opportunity for me to uncover many things, but most pertinent to the CFS recovery was the power of my lower centers, the belly, and forces from the navel down.

I learned that I had a huge amount of repressed rage that kind of turned in on itself and definitely played into the CFS crashing that was happening when I began IST. I had about a year of letting my facilitators lead me into that massive ball of pent-up fury in my belly, like a pulsing energy of intensity. Usually then I would spend some time thrashing about, kicking cushions and yelling at the top of my lungs, until I really got inside the space of that intensity in my body.

The intensity, rage, and anger had been held inside of me for a long time, so that my body was gripping onto that energy and at times collapsing in on itself. Getting my conscious awareness inside that pulsing ball of fury was liberating every single time. My voice released the energy until I was just pure fire, or water, or just force. My body would then feel as if it was vibrating with life and spread throughout the room, the building, even the whole city. The expansion liberated so much of my being that I was just free, and full of joy. Often, there was a lot of laughter after the release.

One day after class and release as described above, I remember being stopped by the sheer beauty of the magnificent red flowers of an Illawarra flame tree, while walking through the lush forest in the suburb of Lane Cove, right near my house. The red of the flowers and their luxurious fullness were so sensual to me that I just had to stop and wonder at them. I had probably walked past them many times, yet never really noticed them as more than a nice picture. Stopped in that moment, I was immersed in the magnetic vibrancy of the tree's invitation. It touched my belly and my own sensuality, activating and highlighting the vitality that had been released from the day before. I felt part of it and yet also in wonder at the whole scene.

Those days were such a reawakening, coming back into my own life force and re-learning the joy of creating. I was writing for newspapers and magazines, doing freelance journalism from home. I was using the meditation techniques to take on my own business, learning how to navigate through the maze of research and writing without crashing. I was liberated.

The lower centers of energy in the body, which I am calling the belly, are really like the engine for our body of life. Life force is vitality, it is intensity, it is sensual, and it is also vibrant.

Many people, myself included, come to the exploration of these lower centers with a lot of trapped life through the suppression of intense emotions such as anger or rage or even sexual desire. All of those emotions can be like the front face of the underlying trapped vitality in the belly.

Rage, for example, can be a result of trapped life force. Once it flows in a session, where there is a whole structure of safety set up for the client to explore this intense set of feelings, that energy expresses very differently than it does in its trapped form.

Peter Levine with Ann Frederick in the revolutionary book, *Waking the Tiger: Healing Trauma*, talks about trauma as one of "the most important root causes for the form of modern warfare has taken. Traumatic reenactment is one of the strongest and most enduring reactions that occurs in the wake of trauma."[10]

Levine describes the implosion of anger thus:

Like the pigeon that tries frantically to escape, but is recaptured and held prisoner once more, trauma victims beginning to exit immobility (of trauma-related shock) are often trapped by their own fear of abrupt activation and their potential for violence. They remain in a vicious cycle of terror, rage, and immobility. They are primed for full-out escape or raging counter-attack, but remain inhibited because of fear of violence to themselves and others.[11]

My family had a history of emotional violence, as my maternal grandfather was diagnosed with bipolar disorder and had outbursts at times that were extremely impactful to those around him. In addition, the impact of WW2 on both sets of grandparents and the way that was passed onto my

---

10. Peter A. Levine and Chris Sorensen, *Waking the Tiger: Healing Trauma* (Solon, OH: Findaway World, LLC, 2017), 225.

11. Peter A. Levine, *Waking the Tiger,* 103.

parents created a pattern in me of turning in on myself. I even ended relationships because I saw this force was affecting my loved one. I left countries and moved to new cities, unconsciously wanting to be free of the force that I felt hurt those around me, all the time also desperately wanting love.

In those IST sessions on the hot Sydney nights at class, I was able to go towards that same force that had me running all over the world and leaving my loved ones behind. Feeling this ferocity and expressing it safely in a fun environment where everyone enjoyed the release and the wash of vitality it brought, I started to learn that same energy had so much else to offer me.

Entering the pulsing intensity of the rage, I realized this vibrant aliveness in my belly was passionately caring about others, it was intensely creative, and it was full of joy. The terror and rage that had been locked up inside was in fact just the surface of a huge well of energy. And the more that flowed, the more my rage turned into passion.

It turned out that the rage was in fact just energy that had become blocked. Blocked through holding in anger, frustration, intensity. And when it flowed, it became joyful, passionate, and creative wellbeing. I felt alive and inspired when this wellspring of anger was unblocked and the life force was allowed to flow freely.

When I expanded into that oceanic force of intensity, and brought awareness into the nadir of this part of myself, it became untapped potential for giving, for being in states of stillness and presence, for healing.

An important part of IST is the metaphysical dimension that it brings to the psychotherapeutic experience of emotional release. The spiritual awakening that had happened for me as a result of the CFS and traveling in Malawi had a place to really mature and deepen. The techniques brought a precision and amplification of this previously unknown and unmapped territory inside of myself.

Again, there was a stark contrast between this newfound life inside of myself and the stagnancy I had felt as a financial journalist working in Sydney CBD, reporting on stock markets and equities around the world, and then in London writing on European equities. Before I started spiritual exploration, life felt barren to me. After the initial intense challenge of making the pace, learning the trade, getting into the best jobs, and learning to capture stories, there was a chasm of emptiness. Interviews with brokers, analysts, and economists, while often interesting on an intellectual level, were devoid of any real meaning. And I certainly did not have any sense of higher purpose.

I remember hearing that one head broker in the city had just got up from his desk and walked out, never to be seen again. He had friends, family, a whole network of colleagues, and he was an important expert in his field who took calls from journalists every single day. But one ordinary day, he got up from his desk and just walked out. No one saw him again to my knowledge.

When I heard that story, I felt a tinge of sadness but also a huge knowing of why he did it. The emptiness, the chasm of meaningless that is there in watching those numbers go up and down day in, day out, constantly searching for that big win, making the dollars work out.

I remember meeting a man in an investment firm who had retired but still spent his days playing golf with his finance buddies and coming into the office to make comments to young reporters like me. It just felt so deeply sad that this man had nothing else in his life to be passionate about but the office and his finance buddies.

It was unexpected to discover that in fact the emptiness that I felt and the deep anguish in my heart that churned inside of me was in fact a desire to find something with a lot more meaning. I realized that I wanted a sense of spiritual connection, something more than this material reality that we live in most of the time. I was already seeking without knowing it, going to meditation retreats, reading Buddhist texts, speaking with teachers, throwing away all of my stuff, and renouncing my previous life in a somewhat overly hasty attempt at transformation.

Traveling to Africa showed me an entirely different way of seeing the world. Malawi is one of the poorest countries in the world, yet I met some of the sweetest people with huge smiles and warm inviting hearts.

My own heart broke open when I was confronted by a little girl who did not have any money to buy a book to write in, and I had nothing to give her. A young man who wanted to go to school but had to help his dad on the canoe get the fish and take out tourists. I realized how enormously wealthy I had been my whole life just because of the plethora of opportunities that were afforded me by my birth.

I realized that even with very little money in my bank and only the ten pounds sterling in my pocket that I had borrowed from the young men I met on a truck, I was so rich. So unbelievably wealthy compared to these people living by the lake. I have had so much grace in my life, opportunity, and choice. It broke me open.

Yet when I lay there on that mat with Ruth-Helen's hand on my heart, I did not feel any difference between myself and that little girl by the lake with no shoes and a little dress, just wanting a book. In my heart, I felt as if I was a little girl in a cave, with nothing at all, and lost without my family. Abandoned to die alone.

The sense of spiritual presence that landed in the room as I cried for that little girl long ago was vast, deep, and full of light. My heart blew up as if it was made of cosmic spaces filled with stars, illuminating my consciousness with light.

I felt one with myself, with the universe, with all of humanity. As if I had come home.

Samuel Sagan wrote in the introduction for his book *Regression Past-Life Therapy For Here and Now Freedom:*

> *Regression is one of the great techniques of the future in the fields of self-discovery and psychotherapy. One of its essential characteristics is that it integrates two dimensions within the same process: a psychotherapeutic dimension, and a metaphysical one.*
>
> *To psychotherapists, regression is a transpersonal technique allowing explorations and releases of unprecedented depth, and through which a much needed metaphysical dimension can be incorporated into psychotherapy.*
>
> *To spiritual seekers, regression is a major tool in the opening of perception, a powerful awakener of the third eye, and above all a path of mental de-conditioning. It achieves a profound and systematic purification of the emotional layer—not unlike the catharsis which Bernard de Clairveaux, patron of the Templars, used to describe with the Latin word defæcatio, considering it an indispensable preliminary to higher spiritual experience.[12]*

Sagan goes on to explain that regression, which is part of IST, aims at exploring and releasing emotional blockages and mental complexes, specifically reaching hidden subconscious and unconscious memories.

---

12. Samuel Sagan, *Regression: Past-Life Therapy for Here and Now Freedom* (Roseville, N.S.W: Clairvision, 1996), 1.

> *Even in the first sessions, it is not uncommon to experience flashbacks that cannot be related to any experience in this life, but are accompanied by a deep feeling and an inner certitude that they refer to yourself. Hence the name 'past-life therapy' is often given to regression.*[13]

That was true for me, since my first session was deeply profound and clearly what would be termed a past life. And it did not matter that I did not believe in past lives either. It still unfolded just as it needed for me to have a big release, and connect with parts of my heart that were previously hidden.

Ruth-Helen mirrored that drive for spiritual connection back to me, telling me that I was clearly looking for more than therapy, but was on a path of searching for transformation. I knew it was true when she said it. My actions for the last two years were clear evidence, but I had not really thought of myself like that at all. Perhaps because the circles I had previously moved through viewed spiritual seeking as vague, wishy-washy, and even a bit weird.

It is understandable that spiritual seekers are seen this way among many rational people, because in the world of spiritual seekers there is so much deception and delusion that it pushes away those of us who value intellect and grounded logic. There are lots of people who take the whole area of spirituality as just another way to make big money and manipulate people, using the values of materialism to take

---

13. Ibid.

advantage of people's real seeking for something greater. There are others who naively believe that just being a good person and giving out 'good vibes' is enough. For people like me, it definitely is not.

In that moment in Ruth-Helen's office in Chatswood, Sydney, I could feel the truth of it. The truth of being a spiritual seeker felt for me like being someone on a quest for meaning. I wanted to break through the illusions, the greed, the world of illusion that I had glimpsed in myself and in the world around me so far.

I had traveled around the world, meeting so many people, and I had succeeded in the media career that I fought so hard for, only to find out it was just another version of the treadmill. When I had the husband, the cute apartment, the well-paid job in London, UK, I could feel the loneliness that was inside of me. I was disillusioned. I thought this emptiness was separate from the CFS, and perhaps it was, but also perhaps it was not.

No matter how disillusioned I became with the heaviness of the illness and the lack of meaning in my life, I never wanted to give up. I wanted answers and I wanted help to find them inside of myself.

BECOMING THE HEALER
– THE GREATEST GIFT OF ALL

Nothing in my life before I had CFS prepared me for the wondrous journey of discovery through IST. Seeing my clients' inner worlds with clarity and recovering from things that had previously seemed insurmountable was so gratifying.

I have rarely been bored because I was lucky enough to have an unusually vivid life. I have traveled around the world since I was a baby, met interesting people, been inspired by beautiful and terrible places that expanded my horizons. As a competitive swimmer in my teens, I won races in front of cheering crowds, explored the delights of relationships and sexuality with partners from different walks of life, even immigrated several times, and started two different careers working full-time in four different cities, across three continents.

Still, I was being blown open when I started to immerse myself in the IST trainings. There were many things that I uncovered about my own depths, bringing the light of self-awareness into places where there was none, but there were even more in learning to facilitate the ignition of self-awareness for others.

I also met and was able to work with many people who had severe issues of fatigue, burnout, CFS, and even more recently people with Long COVID.

One of my earliest clients who had CFS was part of my inspiration to be an IST practitioner. Sofia was 21 years old and very weighed down by a dark cloud of CFS when she first came to see me for IST in Australia. This was a young woman with the kind of intensity that blasted through her dark eyes. She asked probing questions throughout the whole week. She was vegan and deeply concerned about any spiritual work where people were not vegetarian, vehemently arguing her point that this was the right path. She was passionate about everything in her life, but she also struggled with incredibly bad migraines, gut issues, and debilitating fatigue.

Sofia stood out to me, because of the way her presence filled the room and the intensity with which she dove into the techniques. She was using IST to work on a lot of early childhood trauma including sexual abuse in her family. The sessions were largely used for finding the underlying or hidden sources of samskaras. The word *samskara* is an ancient Indian Sanskrit word roughly translated as emotional wound or scar, which is the real source of suffering.

We all have deeply imprinted memories that repeat themselves, influence the way we see the world, and condition our behavior and experiences. These are samskaras. Michael Singer says,

> *In the yogic tradition an unfinished energy pattern is called a Samskara. This is a sanskrit word meaning "impression," and in the yogic tradition it is considered*

> *one of the most important influences affecting your life. A Samskara is a blockage, an impression from the past. It's an unfinished energy pattern that ends up running your life... A Samskara is a cycle of stored past energy patterns in a state of relative equilibrium. It is your resistance to experiencing these patterns that causes the energy to keep cycling around itself.[14]*

One of the differences between Singer's approach and IST is that in IST there is an interactive component of exploration, and the goal is to really see the source of the blockage, together with your practitioner. Essentially, the practitioner will lead the client into an inner space of consciousness through a meditation-style technique to explore the blockage and find the true source, where a great release happens, beyond what the ordinary mind can comprehend.

In his book *Regression Past-Life Therapy for Here & Now Freedom*, Sagan describes the fundamental mechanism of a samskara:

> *You have a car accident at a particular place. Then, for a long while, each time you drive past that place you feel uneasy; a wave of fear arises. You may even feel uncomfortable*

---

14. Michael A. Singer, *The Untethered Soul: The Journey beyond Yourself* (Oakland, CA: Noetic Books, Institute of Noetic Sciences, New Harbinger Publications, Inc, 2013), 82-83.

just by thinking of the episode. The traumatic imprint left in your mind after the accident is called a samskara. The malaise that subsequently appears each time you drive past the place is called a reactional emotion, or more simply an emotion. The tendency of the samskara to generate a wave of fear whenever remembering the accident is called the dynamism of the samskara.

Basically, all samskaras operate in the same way. Simple. Yet, according to the Upanishads, the final chapters of the Vedas, as soon as the last knot of samskaras in the heart has been untied, the highest state of consciousness is cognized, absolute freedom is reached, and martyo 'mrto bhavati, "the mortal becomes immortal." (Katha-Upanishad 6.15 and Brihad-Aranyaka-Upanishad 4.4.7.)[15]

I still remember leaning over Sofia while she howled with her full open voice at its most intense, expressing the deeply held pain, grief, rage, hurt about some awful childhood events involving her father. Blockages she had carried with her through her whole life unburdening right in front of me. She screamed and cried until it was all lifted and she could feel that little girl inside of herself, vulnerable, light, and tender.

---

15. Samuel Sagan, *Regression: Past-Life Therapy for Here and Now Freedom* (Roseville, N.S.W: Clairvision, 1996), 6.

Once she had really let go, Sofia dropped into a hush, feeling depths inside of herself that she had never consciously experienced before. A huge stillness landed in the room. Even though it was not my own emotional release, I was deeply moved too. My heart felt ripped open and new.

Most importantly, though, Sofia went on to release a lot of very intense grasping, anger, pain, and bitterness that had been left over from the events of her childhood. Years of holding down the immense betrayal, hurt, and rage she felt about these events had weighed down her natural enthusiasm. It not only impacted her emotionally, but also obstructed the innate flow of her vital energies. As she recovered that flow, the vibrant energy of her core nature started to return and she was able to consciously bring it to everything in her life, recovering from the extreme fatigue.

The weightlessness and radiance that shone through her eyes at the end of the course was inspiring to all of us around her. Several years later I learned she had become a physics professor, leading the field with her publications, discoveries, and brilliant ideas.

Helping this young woman to release some of those heavy weights that she had carried since she was very small was liberating for me too. I felt washed and enlivened.

Since then I have spent over 20 years as an IST practitioner completing thousands of sessions for people all over the world, I have continued to feel renewed every single time I am able to help uplift a person out of their blockages and free them of unnecessary energetic burdens.

4

DISCOVERING THE CRASH & THE ROAD TO RECOVERY

As I started to recover through releasing these unwanted emotional blockages, the next step that was pivotal to my own full recovery was understanding the mechanisms behind the crash or collapse in my body of energy.

The crash was actually causing a lot of the CFS symptoms. This was so key to my ability to really get better, because in my experience, until I really knew the true cause, it was really difficult if not impossible to completely address it and change it.

Do you know what it is like to have an energetic crash or a collapse?

The crash is where your energy or vitality just seems to drop through the floor, and you are left feeling like there is less than nothing left. You don't know where all of your life force went, and if you push through the emptiness and fatigue, then symptoms just get worse and worse.

That was one of the main things I had to address in my own journey and then helped many others to overcome.

When I first learned about the importance of understanding and addressing crashing for many people with CFS, it was an early session with Ruth-Helen in her light-filled office in Chatswood, Sydney. Ruth-Helen explained that in my case, and the case of many others with debilitating experience of CFS, regression and releasing stuck emotion was important, but it was not enough to cure the illness.

The cause of the CFS had more to do with something structural in my energy that was crashing or collapsing and triggering many of my symptoms. This needed direct cultivation and strengthening through a set of energetic exercises called "uplifting" that I could practice many times a day.

Immediately after Ruth-Helen explained crashing, I could relate it to my own experiences.

This term crashing described a punctual internal sense of descending heaviness, gripping pain, foggy head, deep, bone-aching fatigue, nausea, stomachaches, newly emerging intolerance to countless foods, and the ensuing reactivity. This plunging into pain and deep fatigue seemed to switch on and off for no apparent reason. At times it drove me crazy with frustration trying to figure it out.

Prior to meeting Ruth-Helen, I had spent a lot of time trying to work out what had caused my own crashes. Did I get too exhausted at the cinema? Did I overdo it at the shopping mall or the party? Did I eat something that triggered a reaction of some kind?

I ruled out foods, entertainment, all sorts of activities that I thought must have made me crash. I was convinced that I had insane food sensitivities, which may have been at least partially true.

Essentially, a crash felt like a collapse. I would be going along fine, doing the things that I really wanted to do, and then suddenly without warning, I started having these violent, heavy symptoms that brought me down.

The sickness would come on within a matter of a few hours, and then last for anything between days and weeks. Sometimes the crash would be dramatic, like the time I was on the way to work on a train and crippling pain started to grip my head at the same time as a violent wave of nausea, so intense that I had to jump off at the next stop to vomit.

Sometimes it seemed to take a few days, beginning with mild nausea, then a night of sleeplessness and restlessness, followed by aching sinuses. Within a few days, I was in bed for a week or more.

Lying down did not always help. Sometimes it seemed to make it worse. I learned to sit and meditate through the pain, breathing gently into the gripping in the quiet darkness of my room.

I was prescribed migraine medication which frankly also made me feel worse, intensifying the nausea without relieving the pain.

The key for me was that there was such a distinct up-and-down pattern in my symptoms. I would be desperately uncomfortable, and then crash, and then recover so that everything would be fine for a while. And the cycle would repeat itself pretty regularly.

For instance, there was one meditation retreat which was two weeks of silence with women in Wales. The first few days were fraught with tension, stomach pain, extreme discomfort, and at times downright anxiety. The agitation in my body was so intense that at the end of the day, I would lie on the floor with my legs on my bed, just waiting for everything to settle until I could sleep.

Then after the first few days, in one particularly long silent (and for me tortured) sit, my stomach gurgled very loudly. Internally, I was sent into fits of silent laughter. It was all I could do to stop myself from laughing out loud.

At that point, I was able to let go, and a huge stillness descended around me for the rest of the retreat. States of what the Buddhists call bliss.

After those days of bliss, returning home on the train, I immediately started to notice the return of the headaches, the extreme discomfort after eating food, the swampy states of inexplicable fatigue, and the aching heaviness in my body. By the time I got to my destination a day later, I was dragging my body to bed like a sack of potatoes.

More and more I observed a general pattern. While on retreat, my symptoms would go through some kind of crescendo to a kind of crash, then I would go into the bliss state, and then upon return from the retreat, I would collapse again into the symptoms. I was still not diagnosed with CFS at that time.

When I got to Sydney over a year after starting to meditate and almost six months later took the course with Ruth-Helen, I realized that what I was experiencing had to do with subtle bodies.

HOW DOES A CRASH RELATE TO SUBTLE BODIES?

Starting with the sense of how this crash in the subtle bodies works from the inside out might help you to see if you can also relate to it, as this is not just an intellectual concept. Maybe you have this visceral felt experience of your own body of energy crashing or collapsing at punctual times for no known reasons.

Samuel Sagan, MD, describes subtle bodies in the *KT Subtle Bodies, the Fourfold Model.*

Human existence does not only consist of maintaining a physical body! Human beings are alive. They experience emotions. They think. And they are capable of self-awareness. These various functions correspond to different layers or vehicles, called subtle bodies.

This is where the orthodox scientific perspective differs from not only the Indian tradition but from virtually all spiritual traditions, whether Eastern or Western. To a twentieth-century materialist, all functions performed by a human being can be explained by the chemistry of the physical body. Life is the product of sexual cells. Thinking is the product of the brain. Awareness is another function of the nervous system, and so on. Whereas Hindus, Buddhists and various Western esotericists maintain that if we can think, for instance, it is because we are endowed with a particular vehicle—a subtle body—which is not made of physical matter, and in which thoughts take place. In the Clairvision model, this vehicle is the astral body. From this perspective, the function of the brain is not to 'secrete' thoughts, but to receive thoughts from the astral body. The brain acts as a mirror, and not as the generator of thought processes.[16]

---

16. Samuel Sagan, MD, *KT Subtle Bodies, the Fourfold Model*, Point Horizon Institute. 2011, written PDF for the audio recorded online correspondence course, 33.

Let's use this context to examine what I am calling a crash or a collapse in the subtle bodies. Firstly, lots of people experience a very minor version of the crashing mechanisms without even realizing it.

For example, say you were on a really long Zoom meeting. While you felt light and vibrant when you got onto the call, you increasingly felt heavy, fatigued, and even got a headache towards the end of it.

Or when you were involved in an unfortunate and deeply ugly family argument, where perhaps you felt good before you attended that event, but after the argument had broken out, you left feeling kind of physically awful. Perhaps you felt heavy, or cloudy or even had a headache, or nausea, in contrast to the vibrancy and aliveness that you had felt before you entered your family home that day?

Or what about that day that you spent at the mall with some friends, and while you had a great day, you got home totally exhausted feeling as if you had run a marathon? Even though you were so deeply fatigued, it was difficult to sleep because you felt stimulated and buzzed from the day's event, and then there was a kind of hangover feeling for the next few days?

Or what about when you had a huge emotional reaction about something. You really went for it and expressed your sadness, rage, anger, upset-ness, but at the end of it you felt terrible, as if your head became a wet soggy blanket?

Some people describe this feeling as being "dumped," alluding to a heaviness from above as if a garbage truck had just unloaded its trash on their head. They were up, and then for some reason, they got "dumped" and their energy was down. It doesn't feel good for a normally well person to get dumped. It is certainly exhausting, but it is nowhere near as dramatic as what happens to someone with CFS "crashing."

People with chronic fatigue of some kind can really crash or collapse when they get dumped, having very serious, debilitating symptoms for weeks, months, or years.

WHY DO PEOPLE GET DUMPED, OR EVEN CRASH?

Energetic or nonphysical experiences are really difficult to describe because our culture does not have an acceptable language for these things. We largely have to speak in metaphor to describe an experience which is not at all vague when you have one yourself.

If you think of everything to do with the life force or vitality as belonging in the area of the body, from head to toe so to speak, it makes sense because we actively feel life in the body.

If you have ever jumped into the ocean and swum in the waves, your body might have felt tingly, alive, open to connecting with the energy of nature. This invigorating feeling of cool water on your skin, the taste of the salt on your tongue, and its sting in your eyes might have seemed to bring the essence of aliveness into your body.

Or if you ever went hiking up a mountain, you might have felt the sheer exhilaration of reaching the top. It was hard work, and you were tired, but at the same time, there was a sense of the clarity in the air, the vibrancy of the landscape around you, the freshness in your head, and the levity of being alive so intense that you could touch it.

These experiences of life are easy to spot for most of us. Yours might not be exactly the same as the ones described above, but you can spot the similarities—the feeling of aliveness, the connection with nature, the exhilaration in your body that feels good.

In contrast, walking through Times Square in New York City, or riding the packed subway in Tokyo, or lining up in a long hour to check in at the airport among throngs of people, tend to make us feel squeezed, dense, heavier, buzzy. These things leave us stimulated, but in a different way. Stimulated in a way that is more contracted, contained, busy, and even draining. It is not the same as being physically exhausted from exercising in nature. It is as if we were drained from the emotional and energy buzz of the city rather than our interaction with nature. It feels different.

Being on a busy subway, traveling through a packed airport, walking in the buzz of city lights and throngs of people moving to and from their destinations, getting stuck in hours and hours of traffic can cause dumping of some kind, even if you are not really doing much. After all, it is not like hiking up a mountain. You are just catching a train, walking through the square, getting to your flight on time, mundane tasks that do not take a lot of physical exertion, nor are they intellectually challenging. Yet they are somehow exhausting.

The energy in those examples is that of the stimulation of the level of consciousness, or thoughts, and emotions. I am not saying that the stimulation of thoughts and emotions is bad, more that there is a need for a balance of some kind between the life force energy and consciousness.

Think of it as two poles, consciousness and life. We move between them every day, and in reality they are both part of our experience all of the time. They are like two ends of a spectrum of our experience. Sometimes we are more in the life aspect of the experience—in nature, while having sex, in the morning when quietly taking a few minutes to wake up. Other times we are more at the consciousness end of the spectrum—busy, stimulated by our phones, our screens, the city lights, multiple demands from the people in our lives at home and at work, and the loudness of our emotional reactions, even if it is just a minor bout of road rage.

We move through these two aspects of our experience every day, all day, consciousness and life. And while ideally we are meant to have some kind of balance inside of ourselves, in reality most often this harmony is absent. One aspect of this imbalance between life and consciousness inside of us is that many people get dumped, and some people crash. This disharmony inside of our own selves leads to much agitation, including issues with sleep, discomfort, pain, disease, and even illness.

The subtle bodies of human beings have changed a lot in the last 150 years. When I use the term subtle bodies, what I mean is that human beings are not just physical, but also have more subtle aspects to them: life force, a mind, and a spiritual or higher self. In fact, I would go further to say that our consciousness, our whole being is made of subtle bodies.

We have undergone globalization, information overload, and the fast-paced change of technology. And while all of this has been happening around us, it has changed our inner landscape of consciousness too.

"In 1900, just under 40 percent of the total US population lived on farms, and 60 percent lived in rural areas," according to economist Jayson Lusk, Vice President and Dean of the Division of Agricultural Sciences and Natural Resources (OSU Agriculture) at Oklahoma State University. *"Today, the respective figures (living on farms and rural areas) are only about 1 percent and 20 percent,"* Lusk says in his blog, *The Evolution of American Agriculture*, published June 27, 2016.[17]

It is easy to see from these statistics that people in the past were far more grounded in the land, and in nature than they are now. Nature was part of their lives. I always think

---

17. Jayson Lusk, "The Evolution of American Agriculture," Jayson Lusk, June 27, 2016, http://jaysonlusk.com/blog/2016/6/26/the-evolution-of-american-agriculture.

of my own great-grandparents who were market farmers in London, UK and never saw the ocean in their whole lives even though they lived to be in their 80s. And my great-grandparents on the other side of the family were extremely unusual for their time because they took three months to sail across the ocean to emigrate from the UK to Malawi in Africa so that my great-grandfather could pursue his career as a botanist. And even as immigrants, they were also totally connected to nature in a way that no one alive in my family is now.

When I was studying directly with Samuel Sagan, in White Cliffs, NSW in Australia, we had many fascinating discussions about the changes in the modern world and how it has impacted our subtle bodies and consciousness. We talked often about how fast human consciousness has developed and changed over the last 100 years.

Sagan was clear that,

Change is a key word of the modern Western world. Only 100 years ago, people rarely changed jobs or partners. Go back another one or 200 years, and you would find that in many tasks, people followed the model of their parents. From one generation to the next, the modus operandi of practical life didn't vary much. Now, change has become a constant fact of life. The speeding up of technological progress is such that every few years, entire fields of professional activities undergo major transformations.[18]

The fast pace of change in technology, globalization, and science are all relatively new things that strengthen, stimulate, and even inflame the consciousness end of the spectrum of the human experience.

At the same time, our life force energy is increasingly under attack and unsupported by the environment or food, as it once was. We are less and less connected to nature, the environment around us is increasingly polluted, climate change is hitting the Earth with more and more disasters, processed food is the norm, and everything that we eat is markedly less nutritious than it was 150 years ago.

As a result of this strengthening of consciousness and the weakening of our life force, there is an imbalance in our subtle bodies. This creates an apparent conflict between the poles of life and consciousness, even though these two poles are always part of our experience in one way or another. We never experience one of these poles without the other, yet they now seem to be disharmonious.

This disharmony in our subtle bodies can create issues with sleep, digestion, increased neuroticism, headaches, allergies, and a myriad of other symptoms.

---

18. Samuel Sagan, MD, *KT FuXi's Mountain*, Point Horizon Institute. 2011, written PDF for the audio online correspondence course, 126. Quoted with the kind permission of Dr. Samuel Sagan in 2007.

We get dumped, we crash, we get sick a lot because our life energy is depleted, and our consciousness is overstimulated. In essence the consciousness side of the pole is dominating our life energy.

Common sense might say, well, let's eat organic food, or even grow it ourselves, move away from the cities into pristine natural environments, and just eradicate technology and any other stressors. Unfortunately, that is not practical, and it does not solve the problem on an individual level, let alone a global level.

I have moved out of cities and changed my diet many times. I have embraced nature and run away from stress. It did help my symptoms for a short time, but never took away the illness completely. In fact, early on in my journey with CFS, quitting everything seemed to make me sicker.

When you have tried all the physical approaches available and they are not facilitating a cure, then it is time to ask yourself: is there an energetic component to the illness I am experiencing?

Of course diet is important as food is generally pretty crap in the current Western world. And there is definitely a need for people to get more time in nature, and to do slow, gentle incremental steps to return to exercise as part of the recovery. There are approaches to the gut, sorting out the environment of the digestive system. And addressing any underlying issues from the virus or parasites that you have caught that triggered this illness in the first place.

But then if there is still a set of symptoms that involves heavy ongoing, unexplained fatigue, and you do not know why, perhaps it is time to look at what is needed on the level of subtle bodies.

CASE STUDY – MARIA RECOVERY FROM EXECUTIVE BURNOUT AND CFS

Maria was 53 years old when she came to a weekend meditation workshop that I ran in Boston, Massachusetts in 2010. She had been diagnosed with CFS and burnout, after her health took a dive when she was in a top executive marketing position at a Fortune 500 company in the USA. Maria was a Rhodes Scholar, immensely talented and bright. But when she first came into the room on that weekend, her short brunette curly bob looked flat, her eyes a little dull, and her mouth kind of tight.

The amazing thing was that, as the weekend progressed, Maria just brightened up more and more with every single exercise that we did. By the end of the weekend, she was shining and bubbly, sharing with the group how much she had received from all the exercises that we did.

Maria was so responsive because we did a lot of activities that weekend that were directly aimed to help her learn to uplift her energy above. She learned how to use the practices to avert any crashing and heavy dumping in her life force and return to her levity of being for herself.

She was a very quick learner, but more than that, Maria's energy was so responsive to the techniques because it was what she needed at that time. She had been sick for a couple of years, and looking for treatments that might help her recovery. Even Maria was surprised how much this style of meditation and the uplifting techniques contributed to her vitality and clarity of mind.

I realized that weekend that you will see pretty quickly, in about six to eight hours of techniques or a workshop, whether or not these exercises are going to work for you. The results speak for themselves. It is not necessarily for everyone, but for those who do find it works, it will be clear within a few sessions or one short weekend.

Maria then did have to go through a process of learning to bring that levity into her own life, and how to make it really work for herself. Like any new type of exercise, it took some months for her to apply it at this level but she was highly motivated because it had worked for her on the weekend, and she could see that it was possible.

5

CENTERS OF ENERGY ABOVE THE HEAD, LEAKING, AND CFS

Even when you are starting to get better, and in what I would call the second phase of CFS, a crash can appear to come out of the blue, taking you by complete surprise when you thought everything was going great.

Once the trajectory towards recovery is engaged, the crashes are shorter in duration, and the space between them extends in time.

It might seem strange to you that extreme symptoms like headaches, flu-like symptoms, nausea, vomiting, belly aches, and diarrhea can flare sometimes for what seems like no reason at all.

If you are someone who is impacted by the energetic side of CFS, then sometimes those crashes occur because blockages or stuck energies wreak havoc punctually.

A trip to the mall, a party with friends, or a long business conference or series of Zoom meetings can result in a three weeks in bed, making you feel the need to withdraw from the world just to avoid the dreaded crashing.

Or it may be just as confounding when a long family gathering, where there is a lot of unspoken emotional tension and history in the air, relegates you to bed with aching bones and a sick belly for a couple of days.

The so-called "good" emotions can be just as intense and leave you laid out for days too. Like extreme joy or exhilaration. I once had a massive crash after jumping out of a plane on a parachuting trip with friends. I laughed with so much intensity once I was out of that plane and coasting like an eagle high above that I crashed badly and spent the night with a terrible migraine, vomiting my guts up.

Maybe you even use the term *crash* when something like this happens because it is just such a good onomatopoeic word to describe what happens. A lot of people do use this term precisely because of the evocative way it describes exactly how it feels to go down with a bout of CFS and some kinds of burnout.

As I said before, CFS and burnout can be triggered by more than one thing, so for a whole group of people in these categories, a crash can also have to do with a leakage in the subtle bodies where the centers of energy that are above the head fall into the energy of the body. I will explain this as simply as I can.

Just as we have centers of energy pertaining to the physical body, like the third eye, the heart and the sexual centers, we also have energy above the head and below the body.

Crashing really happens from the energy above.

When I had CFS and began to learn about crashing and dumping from Ruth-Helen, the first step was to see what was happening for myself, instead of just believing what she or anyone else told me. For quite a few months, I was still pretty skeptical about it all, yet I wanted to give it a go, and so I continued to attend IST sessions with Ruth-Helen to see what she could help me to know about my own subtle-body mechanisms of crashing.

It took me some time in the sessions to see how I was really crashing from above. I realized that sometimes when I was collapsing, I would feel like a huge weight was coming down on me and that I was under a dark cloud. In contrast when I was really well, I felt light, bouncy, alive, and uplifted.

After a few sessions with Ruth-Helen, I began to see how the subtle energies were working when I crashed, seeing the movement between feeling vital and bouncy to falling into the crash with finer and finer levels of observation. This refined vision or knowing of the way I moved between the vital state and the crashed state was the key to recovery for me.

At first, it was like falling over when you are ice skating. I was up, and then I was down, and there was no or very little awareness of the transition at all. But as I refined my awareness, I began to see that there was an in between when the heaviness would start to gather above and the potential for a crash was looming.

I remember saying to Ruth-Helen, "How am I ever going to see the crash before it happens? That seems impossible!"

Sitting opposite me, looking deeply into my eyes, her enthusiasm shining through, she replied, "You are nearly there. Just the fact that you are asking that question is already a step towards seeing. Keep looking and you will see."

It took a few more weeks after that conversation, but I did develop the ability to sense and prevent the crashing more and more often, until it became part of my conscious awareness all the time.

When I started to sense the collapse for myself, I was at my sister's house. It was not in an IST session but in my daily life, with my sister, her husband, and child, several hours north of Sydney. I was helping with the toddler and the housework when all of a sudden I started to sense the beginning of pain, but it was above my head. It felt like a bunch of rocks, and it was painful. I recognized the pain because I had felt it in my body many times before.

I stepped outside to call Ruth-Helen on the phone, and she talked me through a few brief yet effective systematic exercises to bring me back to sealing my system. The call was probably no longer than 10 minutes. I was standing outside my sister's place, looking up at the dark green trees reaching up into the deep blue sky. The smoke lifted up out of me, and I did not get the headache; the pain went away. That is when I became very motivated to practice those exercises many times a day.

Sagan explains this phenomenon of the collapse for people with CFS in his *Knowledge Track Flow of Life*.

In the KT Flow of Life section 2.4, Sagan talks about how some people with CFS/ME are experiencing an imbalance in intensity of "astral" forces above the head, draining the life force or "etheric."

In Sagan's model, the term *astral body* refers to the vehicle of emotions and thoughts. Incidentally, the same term is used by Austrian Rudolf Steiner, the founder of anthroposophy, leading to many innovative ideas still used today such as Waldorf education, biodynamic agriculture, and anthroposophical medicine.

> *The astral body is the vehicle of the mind (manas in Sanskrit). In the Clairvision mapping, the terms 'mind' and 'astral body' are used interchangeably. ...The astral body of the Clairvision mapping can also be equated with that of Indian masters. Indian masters commonly use*

the term astral body to refer to the sukshma sharira of Vedantic classification.[19]

Someone with CFS/ME who has the crashing or collapsing of the column above will usually have a high degree of astral intensity in the centers above their head.

There is a type of CFS person who tends to respond really well to the Clairvision techniques, and that is the kind with a certain kind of density, intensity, or dynamism in the subtle-body structures above the head. That intensity and structure above can sometimes result in the whole thing collapsing into their life force and physical body, making them very unwell.

Many times, Dr. Sagan told me personally of my own subtle bodies, that this intensity in my own column above belongs above, and not in the body of life force. He used the term "etheric" for the vehicle of life force.

"The etheric body can be equated with the prana-maya-kosha, 'envelope made of prana' of the Hindu tradition, and with the qi (also known as chi) of the Chinese tradition."[20]

---

19. Samuel Sagan, *A Language to Map Consciousness*, Clairvision School, accessed June 11, 2024, https://clairvision.org/books/altmc/a-language-to-map-consciousness.html.

20. Samuel Sagan MD, *A Language to Map Consciousness*, Clairvision School, accessed June 11, 2024, https://clairvision.org/books/altmc/a-language-to-map-consciousness.html.

Dr. Sagan shared with me a number of times about a case study of a woman who saw him for IST sessions because she was regularly spending three weeks in bed with CFS crashes:

Her column of Spirit was quite crystallized. But that day, something quite dramatic was happening in her subtle bodies. It was as if her column of Spirit was too heavy for her to hold. It was literally collapsing into her head. So badly that her etheric was unable to retain its integrity.

Imagine a mule carrying bags of stones and collapsing to the ground under their weight. It is about what this woman's etheric felt like.[21]

Sagan says that the patient came to him one day just as a crash was about to happen and the energies above were "collapsing into her head." It was so bad that her life force was unable to retain its integrity, he says.

I was blown away when I first read his words: *"Imagine a mule carrying bags of stones and collapsing to the ground under their weight."*

That description really jumped out at me as the image was exactly what I had experienced myself when I had CFS.

Working with this one CFS patient who was regularly crashing to the point that she would need three weeks in bed,

---

21. Samuel Sagan MD, *KT FuXi's Mountain*, Point Horizon Institute, 2011, written PDF for the audio online correspondence course, 121. Quote used with the kind permission of Dr. Samuel Sagan in 2008.

Samuel was able to avert the crisis before it happened. So, the first thing Samuel did was to pull up energies in her column of Spirit. He uplifted the stones, so to speak.

> *It did not involve any medications, remedies or the pressing of any gateways or points on the body—simply the uplifting power of consciousness. He got her to close her eyes, and he pulled. It only took a minute or two.*
>
> *Then something quite spectacular took place. The woman opened her eyes and said, "It's gone. The attack is gone. The headache is much better already. I'm not feeling tired."*
>
> *That was hard to believe. Five minutes earlier she was a complete wreck. She had to drag herself to the appointment. She had a screaming headache and cramp-like pains in her muscles. There was a thick cloud in front of her eyes. She wasn't completely there. And she was convinced she was going to have to stay in bed for three weeks, as had been the case several times in the past after an attack of this kind.[22]*

This story was very inspiring for me at the time of my recovery, and as a result a big part of getting better for me was learning to implement those exercises for myself, and that came with engaging a whole system of training. It began

---

22. Ibid. Quote used with the kind permission of Dr. Samuel Sagan in 2008.

with Ruth-Helen in her office in Sydney, but then I joined the classes at the Clairvision School, learning to build my subtle bodies and develop inner vision, and later trained directly with Samuel Sagan himself.

It is one thing for a practitioner or a healer to do the exercises for you, or even to talk you through it so that you can do them together, but quite another to learn how to shift out of a crash for yourself. This is something that happens with practice and over time as it requires increasing subtle levels of strength and agility where you did not have them before.

I would like to use the analogy here of weight training. If you start weights at the gym and your trainer gives you some new exercises that works out a muscle that you never consciously used before, you start to really feel that part of your body in a way that you did not before. At first, it might be a bit difficult because there is no awareness there. It could be hard to separate out from nearby muscles or even a bit numb. Then you might have pain because the muscle is protesting at being used with the weights. Finally, it becomes integrated, and you can use that muscle when you want or need to.

What differs from weight training is that cultivating subtle bodies in this way has a spiritual element, just because the subtle bodies include this aspect of ourselves. The intention of developing the subtle bodies through regular exercises is really to connect to the higher self, the spiritual aspect of our consciousness which is loosely speaking self-awareness and perhaps also the pathway to our own inner peace.

That's why training in this style of work was something of a wonderful adventure for me. A whole new phase of my life that involved traveling through inner worlds and making huge discoveries that did lead to my recovery from CFS and so much more. I became a spiritual seeker who was finding what I was looking for, real in-depth experiences of inner peace, spiritual fire, heart opening, and getting to know myself at the level of being.

This is a journey that takes you inside of yourself, understanding deeper aspects of your consciousness and body of life force. Learning to cultivate your own subtle bodies in a way that fosters the healing power of life and vitality.

As Satprem wrote in 1970 for the preface for his book, *Sri Aurobindo or The Adventure of Consciousness:*

> *The age of adventures is over. Even if we reach the seventh galaxy, we will go there helmeted and mechanized, and it will not change a thing for us; we will find ourselves exactly as we are now: helpless children in the face of death, living beings who are not too sure how they live, why they are alive, or where they are going. On the earth, as we know, the times of Cortez and Pizarro are over; one and the same pervasive mechanism stifles us: the trap is closing*

inexorably. But, as always, it turns out that our bleakest adversities are also our most promising opportunities, and that the dark passage is only a passage leading to a greater light. Hence, with our backs against the wall, we are facing the last territory left for us to explore, the ultimate adventure: ourselves.[23]

CASE STUDY - RICHARD AND UPLIFTING

A few years ago as an IST practitioner myself, I worked with Richard, a very dynamic, frustrated, intense 30-year-old cryptocurrency entrepreneur based in El Salvador who had been sick for nearly 10 years. He responded immediately when I talked with him about dumping, making it clear that he understood exactly what I was referring to. It wasn't hard for me to notice that this tall, slim, dark-featured young man was very intense and over-burdened above his head, just as Sagan described earlier in the *Knowledge Track Flow of Life*.

With CFS the etheric body finds itself under the constant, exhausting pressure of astral intensity. This has a lot to do with the modern lifestyle: stress and all sorts of factors that

---

23. Satprem, *Sri Aurobindo, or, the Adventure of Consciousness* (Delhi, Mysore: Mother's Institute of Research and Mira Aditi, 2008).

raise intensity in the astral body. The astral constantly grasps and wears out the etheric, resulting in exhaustion.[24]

I knew that when I worked with Richard, I was going to have to use the technique of uplifting to help him with his recovery just as Sagan describes in the online correspondence course *KT Flow of Life*.

Sagan goes on to say that:

The Clairvision work has very precise strategies to deal with Chronic Fatigue Syndrome. These have to do with the column above, which is cultivated so it can hold and contain astral intensity, without letting astral intensity lapse into the etheric body. One of the key subtle body techniques here is called uplifting. It uses the column above to pull up venomous astral energies out of the etheric. It is about learning new ways of overall management of your energy.[25]

Everything that Richard did, he did intensely and with a lot of grasping. Since he had become ill, Richard had done every kind of cleanse, all types of physical therapy and a lot of healing work before he came to see me. He was, in his

---

24. Samuel Sagan, MD, *KT Flow of Life*, Point Horizon Institute, 2011, from the written PDF for audio recordings on an online correspondence course, 66.

25. Samuel Sagan MD, *KT Flow of Life*, 76.

words, "extremely frustrated" not as much by the huge sums of money that he had spent flying around the world seeing all kinds of specialist practitioners and medical professionals, as by the amount of time that he said he was wasting on trying to get better instead of being able to live the life that he really wanted to live.

Richard really wanted to be a professional basketball player, and had been very good when he was at his prime in his teens. He had shown such promise that it looked possible at that time that he could have been a professional player in America. He was tall, thin, and very athletic. But he had been crippled with these collapses that happened even when doing basic training.

In our first session together, I pointed out to Richard that he was crashing or collapsing his subtle energy above the head, and that this was really draining him at a deep level. He immediately got what I was pointing to. He was kind of arrogant about being very fast to pick up most things in his life, describing himself as "way ahead of the game compared to most people he meets." Being quick to pick up the techniques and comprehend the system behind it is not unusual for someone with the experience of this type of CFS subtle-body crashing.

As soon as I pointed out the crashing mechanism to Richard, I was able to teach him about uplifting. The technique was something that he used alongside the IST sessions to build his vertical muscle and strength so that he could stop the crashing on his own.

In Richard's case, cultivating subtle body fortitude through uplifting was an important part of the recovery. This is the technique that involves pulling up the heavy dumping or crashing fatigue from above. It is a relatively simple exercise that any IST practitioner can teach a client with CFS to do in the sessions and then on their own at home.

I explained to Richard that in the context of the Clairvision model of subtle bodies, many people with CFS crash because they have something energetic that collapses in their system. Just as we have centers of energy (referred to as chakras in the Indian system) in the heart, the belly, at the base of the body, and even in the third eye between the eyebrows, we have energy centers above the head too.

Meeting with his dark piercing eyes, I explained that sometimes these centers above collapse, meaning that there is energy that is meant to be above the head that falls into the energy corresponding to the body and life force. He nodded back, looking almost annoyed that I had to explain it to him at all.

But he did want to know how it worked, so I described how the energy above the head is meant to stay above the head, so when someone either pulls that down unconsciously or it collapses in on them, there is a possibility of some very violent symptoms. This kind of collapse can give people deep body aches, splitting headaches, crushing fatigue. Over time, this grasping can lead to or exacerbate more serious chronic issues. Subtle-body building, including uplifting, is an important pathway back to vertical levity and lightness of being on an energetic level.

To be super clear, IST is all about finding the real source of what is happening. And if the real source is a physical illness or injury, then that must be addressed for the situation to resolve. Often the healing involves also addressing other levels: the physical, etheric (life force), astral (emotional), and spiritual (meaning things like life purpose and sense of truth).

With CFS or burnout-type situations, the source of the problem can be addressed in IST sessions. It is supplemented by applying meditation-based techniques on a daily basis to strengthen and fortify the subtle bodies, as well as to stop crashing altogether.

Subtle-body building is a systematic pathway to bring integrity back into our system. Building these "energetic muscles" or nonphysical strength takes time because, just as you need to go to the gym regularly to build your physical body, you also need repetitive steps to build your nonphysical body.

Incremental steps to building subtle body strength include meditation-based exercises that help you to bring clarity to your energy centers. For example, a regular meditation on the energy center of the third eye in the middle of the forehead or between the eyebrows, alongside practicing the activation of third-eye functionality during your daily life aims to cultivate, clarify, and strengthen the third eye.

The third eye is a starting point for the meditation and healing style of work from Clairvision School because it is a gateway to subtle perception, or the central control panel to manage the body of energy. Just engaging the third eye properly can initiate profound healing for some people, and awaken spiritual perception.

Sagan says, *"The third eye acts as a main switch for the body of energy. By operating the switch, you activate circulations of vibration all over the body."* He goes on to say, *"For present-day human beings, the etheric body is a weak link. It has become so riveted to the physical body that people no longer have any individual perception of it. Therefore, they cannot consciously use it, and it has become dormant and atrophied."*[26]

Richard was engaged in his subtle body-building exercises from the start. He was absolutely vigilant with a daily meditation and uplifting techniques and soon became able to avert a crash or stop the collapsing before it actually happened. He learned to see the signals and sidestep the whole thing with awareness and using the uplifting technique.

---

26. Samuel Sagan MD, *Awakening the Third Eye* (Roseville, N.S.W, Australia: Clairvision, 1997), 78.

RESOURCES FOR YOU GOING FORWARD

If you want to further explore uplifting and the techniques for cultivating your own subtle bodies, you can find an IST practitioner through writing to info@innerspacetechniques.com and do the online correspondence course KT *Flow of Life* available at www.clairvision.org.

Attending a meditation weekend *Awakening the Third Eye* workshop through the Clairvision School is also a great way to learn these techniques.

And a beginner version of the uplifting technique can be found in the book *Awakening the Third Eye* 10.8, Controlling Headaches. The book is available on Amazon and at the Clairvision website.

6

YINYANG FLOW STATES AND RECOVERY

You know that you are starting to get better as months in bed turn into weeks in bed, and then it's just a few days. Along with that, you start to build your strength, perhaps doing little bits of physical activity without crashing. And then you are able to have stretches of weeks of feeling good.

Or at least that was what happened for me. When I started to use the energetic techniques, it was a bit like graded exercise therapy, where I started recovering by building my energetic muscles, doing uplifting and third-eye meditation, as well as releasing a lot of old emotional baggage. Then as I gradually grew stronger, I was back at work crashing one day out of three, and finally, I was able to go weeks without a crash.

When you are also in this phase, where the recovery really starts to take hold, and the crashes get less and less frequent, there is more room to address the fundamental energetic issues behind this suite of illnesses.

Underlying the crashes and many people's experience of burnout, CFS, and some other immune disorders, there is also a more fundamental issue of living from a place of extreme tension, grasping, or pushing which creates a depletion at a very deep level of the body of life force. Addressing this lack of flow can be a key turning point for many people with one of these chronic illnesses and the symptoms of a collapse in the body of life force.

As noted earlier in chapter one, I started to see a crossover in the conditions of CFS, burnout, post-viral fatigue, and even Long COVID over the years of working with and interviewing people about CFS. Not that these conditions are the same thing, but there is a crossover where some people in each of these categories of illness can find recovery through understanding and then learning to directly address the underlying energetic causes of their suffering.

HITTING THE WALL

Burnout is when you hit the wall—but instead of collapsing, or taking a rest, you scale the wall, and just keep going. It doesn't happen because our to-do list gets long, or because we're weak-willed, or because our kids won't go to bed on time. Burnout arrives when every corner of our lives feels unstable, and we convince ourselves that working all the time will fix it.[27]

Burnout was a term coined in 1974 by Herbert Freudenberger when he was working in New York City in a free clinic established by social movement activists as alternatives to the mainstream medical system.

Those of us who work in free clinics, therapeutic communities, hotlines, crisis intervention centers, women's clinics, gay centers, runaway houses, are people who are seeking to respond to the recognized needs of people. We would rather put up than shut up. And what we put up is our talents, our skills, we put in long hours with a bare minimum of financial compensation. But it is precisely because we are dedicated that we fall into a burnout trap.[28]

When Dr. Christina Maslach, a leading pioneer in research on burnout in the early 1980s, was doing her PhD in social work, she found that people in high-stimulation

---

27. Anne Helen Petersen, *Can't Even: How Millennials Became the Burnout Generation* (London: Vintage Digital, 2021).

28. Herbert J. Freudenberger, "Staff Burn-out," Journal of Social Issues 30, no. 1 (January 1974): 159–65, https://doi.org/10.1111/j.1540-4560.1974.tb00706.x.; Douglas Martin, "Herbert Freudenberger, 73, Coiner of 'Burnout,' Is Dead," New York Times, December 5, 1999, sec. 1.

environments like emergency rooms in hospitals are more likely to burn out. Her work published in journals and books like *Burnout: The Cost of Caring* illustrates how to recognize, prevent, and cure burnout syndrome for nurses, teachers, counselors, doctors, therapists, police, social workers, and anyone else who cares about and for people. At that time, Maslach pointed out what causes the feelings of emotional exhaustion, the callous indifference to people's problems, and the sense of inadequacy about one's ability to help and relate to others.

The callous indifference and the inability to help and relate to others is important in many people's experience of burnout because there is an emotional overwhelm. This emotional overwhelm is on the level of the astral body, meaning that there is an overstimulation of astral energies. This overstimulation results in a squeezing of the life force or etheric energies. Therefore, people get very depleted.

When I looked at Maslach's work, it seemed to me that she was implying that it is not the amount of work that burns people out, but the emotional stress. She saw people in emergency departments and immigration law firms who were functional. And it is true that people can be very busy and highly productive without burning out at all if they feel emotionally connected and supported. This is not as easy a distinction to make as it sounds, because there are work environments where attempts are made to create connection, but they are not successful.

Now we are in a time where burnout is on the rise everywhere, as the world itself has become increasingly overwhelming and many more types of workplaces are under-resourced. Not to mention that growing numbers of people working from home leaves workers without any clear sense of boundaries around their personal life.

More recently, burnout has become something that everyone can experience in all kinds of industries. In 2023 hospitality was the industry with the highest rate of burnout according to an article published at gitnux.com and sourced to the online provider of market and consumer date, *Statista*:

> *Hospitality, lodging, and food services have the highest rate of burnout in the world. About 80 percent of those working in this field say their workload was too much to handle. More than 76 percent of respondents in the industrial, medical, and healthcare industries reported having a large percentage of burnt-out staff, according to Statista.*[29]

The current main cause for burnout according to Statista is the fact that people are unable to unplug from work, whether due to an inability to take time off or a lack of clear boundaries between the workplace and home.

---

29. Jannik Lindner, "Must-Know Burnout Statistics [Recent Analysis]," GITNUX, May 27, 2024, https://blog.gitnux.com/burnout-statistics/.

An article in *Forbes* magazine titled, "New Outlook On Burnout For 2023: Limitations On What Managers Can Do" by Bryan Robinson PhD, published Feb 7, 2023, said:

> *Over 4 million American workers quit their jobs each month in 2022. And poor mental health is skyrocketing as 70 percent of the C-suite with the weight of the world—or at least the company—on their shoulders considered quitting to search for a job that responded to their mental health and wellbeing. A recent survey from Slack found that burnout is on the rise globally, most significantly in the US, where 43 percent of middle managers reported burnout—more than any other worker group.*

It went on to say that:

> *Job burnout is both a people killer and a career killer. The World Health Organization (WHO) officially classified burnout as a medical diagnosis, including the condition in the International Classification of Diseases: a syndrome conceptualized as resulting from chronic workplace stress that has not been successfully managed.*[30]

---

30. Bryan Robinson, "New Outlook on Burnout for 2023: Limitations on What Managers Can Do," *Forbes*, September 12, 2023, https://www.forbes.com/sites/bryanrobinson/2023/02/07/new-outlook-on-burnout-for-2023-limitations-on-what-managers-can-do/?sh=6cc56d724343.

The World Health Organization has diagnosed burnout by three symptoms:

Burn-out is defined in ICD-11 as follows:

Burn-out is a syndrome conceptualized as resulting from chronic workplace stress that has not been successfully managed. It is characterized by three dimensions:
- *feelings of energy depletion or exhaustion;*
- *increased mental distance from one's job, or feelings of negativism or cynicism related to one's job; and*
- *reduced professional efficacy.*[31]

FINDING FLOW AS PART OF THE RECOVERY

Recovery from CFS, burnout and other post-viral conditions can be so much about finding the flow as opposed to pushing or forcing or fighting or even struggling in your life and your energy, therefore rebuilding your vitality.

There is a lot of talk about flow among people online today, but they are not always clear what it really is and how

---

31. "Burn-out an 'Occupational Phenomenon': International Classification of Diseases," World Health Organization, May 28, 2019, https://www.who.int/news/item/28-05-2019-burn-out-an-occupational-phenomenon-international-classification-of-diseases.

it can be helpful. I have found it helpful to use the Chinese language of yinyang.[32]

> *"Yin and Yang are the underlying principles of Chinese philosophy and medicine. Good health is believed to come from a balance of Yin (negative, dark, and feminine) and Yang (positive, bright, and masculine)."*[33]

Being a type A person, or someone who has worked hard to achieve your own success, you might tend more towards the yang or more masculine side of consciousness. You are not alone. This is how people have evolved in our current world, and we are all paying the price for it in one way or another.

In this context, masculine and feminine are qualities that all people have within. We have masculine qualities like the warrior inside of us that knows how to get things done,

---

32. In this book I will use the term yinyang, as Robin R. Wang says, "To capture this broad structure, this book will use the term 'yinyang,' rather than 'yin or yang,' 'yin-yang,' or 'yin and yang.' This reflects the Chinese usage, in which the terms are directly set together and would not be linked by a conjunction."

33. Choh-Luh Li, "A Brief Outline of Chinese Medical History with Particular Reference to Acupuncture," Perspectives in Biology and Medicine 18, no. 1 (September 1974): 132–43, https://doi.org/10.1353/pbm.1974.0013; "Chinese Traditional Medicine," U.S. National Library of Medicine, accessed June 11, 2024, https://www.nlm.nih.gov/exhibition/chinesemedicine/yin_yang.html.

and we have feminine qualities, such as the receptive aspects of our energy and consciousness that is more peripheral or subtle in its orientation.

Take a walk through Times Square in New York City at rush hour and you will be pushed and almost dragged along at breakneck speed to the subway station, see cars, lights, hear sounds of the street, and sense the busy stress-filled locals almost running to their next destination. It is easy to see in an environment like this how human consciousness is heavily orientated towards a more yang, creative, or masculine state as opposed to the more yin, receptive, or flowing state.

In the last 150 years or so, humans have tended to value success above all else. To get there, it is accepted that we need to be striving, pushing, forcing, living out our existence in the creative, go-get-'em modes of approaching life. This is opposed to what the Chinese model might refer to as yin states, or receptivity, letting go, turning back inside, resting, feeling as a way of being.

It's easy to see that we are all out of balance as a species. And being out of balance blocks the possibility of any kind of flow where things are done from a state of frictionlessness instead of forcing or pushing.

Chinese philosophy has the formative concept of yinyang, a complex theory going back thousands of years that points among other things to the contradiction and complementarity between two sides. According to Robin Wang:

> *Although yinyang thought may prompt us to think of harmony, interconnection, and wholeness, the basis of any yinyang distinction is difference, opposition and contradiction. Any two sides are connected and related, but they are also opposed in some way, like light and dark, male and female, forceful and yielding. It is the tension and difference between the two sides that allows for the dynamic energy that comes through their interactions. It is also this difference that enables yinyang as a strategy— to act successfully, we must sometimes be more yin and sometimes more yang, depending on the context.[34]*

I want to loosely use this model of yinyang to show that an over-orientation towards the more masculine states leads to a lack of harmony in our consciousness and our body of energy. It is a major contributor to the devastating levels of fatigue that people experience today. An imbalance at a micro level of our daily lives and at the macro level of the whole world has left us increasingly stripped of life in ourselves and on the Earth too.

In my experience, it also leads to more grasping, creating unnecessary struggle.

This is not just a psychological state, but a way of being in our subtle bodies. When we are overloaded with yang

---

34. Robin Wang, *Yinyang: The Way of Heaven and Earth in Chinese Thought and Culture* (Cambridge: Cambridge University Press, 2012), 6.

motion, our subtle bodies get stuck in grasping, much like a tight fist.

Using the yinyang model implies that the feminine and masculine polarities exist in everything, interdependently.

> *According to yinyang thinking, however, the interdependence of opposites does not simply refer to the relativity of our concepts, but also to how things exist, grow and function. One way that interdependence appears most clearly is through the alternation of yin and yang. The sun is the best example of yang—bright, warming, stimulating growth, and giving a rhythm—but when the power of that yang is developed to the extreme, it is necessary for it to be anchored, regenerated, and sustained by the force of yin. The sun must set. Although yang is the obvious, it cannot thrive without attention to yin.*[35]

In my own recovery, an understanding of how to apply these models and enter flow states at will has helped me to change the old pattern of crashing and burnout and step out of the vicious momentum of grasping-induced fatigue.

Dr. Jun Shan writes on *ThoughtCo.*,

> *Yin and yang (or yin-yang) is a complex relational concept in Chinese culture that has developed over thousands of years. Briefly put, the meaning of yin and yang is that*

---

35. Robert Wang, *Yinyang*, p. 8.

the universe is governed by a cosmic duality, sets of two opposing and complementing principles or cosmic energies that can be observed in nature.

...The yin-yang philosophy says that the universe is composed of competing and complementary forces of dark and light, sun and moon, male and female...

...Generally speaking, yin is characterized as an inward energy that is feminine, still, dark, and negative. On the other hand, yang is characterized as outward energy, masculine, hot, bright, and positive.[36]

In the *I Ching or the Book of Changes*—a classic ancient text in Chinese philosophy depicting how consciousness and energy flow through our lives and days—the hexagram number I is "The Creative," and hexagram II is "The Receptive." There are 64 hexagrams indicating the motions, or changes constantly happening in and around us, yet I and II are the creative and the receptive. This is not insignificant that these two motions go first, as they are seen as primary forces in the way the world works. Here in the *I Ching*, these first two lines are masculine and feminine, and seen as complementary forces that go together in all that we do.

In the description of hexagram II The Receptive, *I Ching or the Book of Changes* says:

---

36. Jun Shan, "What Do Yin and Yang Represent?," ThoughtCo, June 7, 2024, https://www.thoughtco.com/yin-and-yang-629214.

> *The attribute of the hexagram is devotion; its image is the earth. It is the perfect complement of The Creative—the complement, not the opposite, for The Receptive does not combat The Creative but completes it. It represents nature in contrast to spirit, earth in contrast to heaven, space as against time, the female-maternal as against the male-paternal.*[37]

Applied to human affairs, this is about the feminine and the masculine principles within each of us, and the interplay of those forces throughout our lives. We sleep, a yin state. Upon waking and during the day, we go out into the world to conquer, which is a yang motion. But even within the day, there are ebbs and flows, times to be in action and times to sit back and rest.

At the heart of my own patterns of crashing, CFS, and tendency to burnout, there was a deep inner conflict around my relationship to the yin self, the spiritual self, the loving self, versus the rational mind that was driven by certain goals and the need to achieve and survive.

Exploring this inner conflict and the need for harmony in my consciousness and energy was something that I did from the inside out. It wasn't through changing behavior although my behavior did change. It was through an exploration of

---

37. Richard Wilhelm, trans., *I Ching or the Book of Changes* (Arkana, 1989), 10.

the changes inside of myself that I learned to listen to what is needed from one moment to the next to stay in this flow.

I found that neither the more feminine and receptive aspect of myself nor the more yang and creative side were wrong, and that harmony could happen with an appreciation of both aspects.

The *I Ching* explains it well, pointing out that *"in itself the Receptive is just as important as the Creative, but the attribute of devotion defines the place occupied by this primal power in relation to the Creative."*[38]

When the receptive is propelled into opposition and struggle against the creative forces inside of us, the *I Ching* says there is an issue. I relate to this in myself. When I push my own body and energy into states of yang or constant drive to productivity, there is a chronic imbalance, resulting in an overload of grasping, debilitating fatigue, and crashing.

Grasping is the nature of consciousness, and flow is the essence of our body of life force or vitality. When we become overloaded with thoughts and emotions, driven to achieve and do, the balance tips and grasping starts to take over. Grasping results in crashing, fatigue, pain, brain fog and so on. This becomes a vicious cycle for some people. It certainly did for me, many times.

To find my own way to that yinyang harmony inside, I had to recognize the difference between being in a state of flow versus being in a state of fighting or trying. I felt pretty

---

38. Richard Wilhelm, trans., *I Ching or the Book of Changes*, 11.

cheated at times that trying so hard, having good intentions was not enough to keep me physically well. Once I accepted this for what it was, finding subtle ways to shift from forcing or pushing into the state of some kind of flow was key to my big-picture recovery.

I don't think it is a coincidence that my own ability to see this imbalance and address it only came when I started to meditate daily. It became crystal clear that even in meditation these conflicts exist for me.

For example, when I spend days or weeks meditating in silence for 8 or even 10 hours a day, initially, the more masculine force pushes the practices, aiming for enlightenment, whipping me into harshness and self-flagellation when I am not "doing well enough with silence." It makes me laugh out loud just to write it because it is the antithesis of what meditation is supposed to be.

The result of that push is pain, grasping, fatigue, and it is unsustainable. Inevitably at some point in a retreat, I would reach a crescendo of grasping that was so intense I felt I could not go on, and then something would kick in, let go, and start to flow.

One year, I was doing three weeks of silent meditation in Australia, and I had pain every single morning that I woke up. That was a pain of a migraine coming on. Every single day, that familiar intense dark cloud would loom, my neck would hurt, and I felt nauseous. But by lunchtime, I was better.

Walking up the little yellow rocky path to the meditation hall, I remember feeling crushed and dark with gripping intense pain, and something inside said, "This is not all there is. There is something else here that is lightness too. Look for the lightness."

As I stepped one foot in front of the other, feeling heavy and hopeless with fatigue, I started to focus on the periphery of my awareness where there was something different. There was a lightness, like the soft blue of the morning sky. There was a breath so sweet that it almost seemed to lift me up. I still felt the gripping pain in my head and the deep sense of empty darkness, but it was not all there was. There was also levity.

That was a turning point for me because I started to realize that I could turn it around. Consciousness has a momentum towards one thing or another. I could actively focus on the lightness, and it would become lighter. I was finding an innate levity in my consciousness, as if every particle could be lifted. I was surprised, but it worked.

Meditation is a way to practice the art of yin-doing or letting go into something of a flow. Yin-doing is a way that I describe what it means to be actively receptive. Once I started to see this for myself, it didn't take long to learn from the inside that I could not force myself into silence and peace. It could only be done through letting go of the driven, pushing states and entering a way of being actively receptive.

Yet at the same time, going too far into the depths of being yin and receptive can become actual sleep, either in life or in meditation. And if I only slept, I did not get better at all. I needed a flow between the yin and yang motions in my energy.

When the feminine receptivity and the masculine fire are in alignment, then the meditative states start to take off. There is clarity and inner wisdom, a knowing of how to navigate the spiritual practice, and something bigger starts to happen. States can emerge that are no longer personal or driven but follow high spiritual experiences into Being-ness.

In life I applied the same principles, not necessarily to be in high spiritual states of being-ness, but to move into a frictionless flow. I got a few things done each day that really made a difference, took breaks when I needed to, and found out what my body of energy or vitality needed so that I could also go into modes of doing that were based in wellbeing.

Doing from a busy space of consciousness can be immensely grasping and draining. Instead remaining in touch with a background sense of your own being, the part that just is and does not exist just to get stuff done, can be grounding, and energizing. It creates a sense of spaciousness within, and an automatic dispersion of tension. It is the yang-doing resting on its feminine polarity of receptivity and stillness within. This is the interplay that creates flow.

VIRTUOUS CYCLE – INCREMENTAL INTERNAL SHIFTS THAT CULTIVATE ALIVENESS WITHIN

Just like I did, you might have already changed your life quite dramatically more than a few times in the attempt to get better. Moved states, countries, radically changed your diet, shifted your career to support your new physical requirements, and more.

For me it took some radical shifts before I really found the way to turn my internal landscapes towards a flow. I didn't immediately recognize that the solution was not so much in changing external situations but in making incremental internal changes in how I managed my energy on a daily basis.

This new way of approaching my own state was about cultivating vital energy rather than draining it. A virtuous cycle rather than a vicious cycle.

The transformation that I needed was inside of myself. It involved learning to see when I went into overdrive, and how to soften and let go without giving up. This is a deep practice that does not come from running away from the things outside that seem to trigger the pain. It comes from something very core of one's self knowing itself. The opposite of ignoring the pain, and yet also not the same as indulging the pain. Opening.

I was in my early twenties when I first came down with CFS, and a few major things were happening in my life that I was ignoring.

Firstly, I had started drinking a lot of alcohol when I was in my teens and also had a lot of antibiotics as a child with many sinus and ear infections. This left my gut biome out of whack and made me sick, giving me irritable bowel syndrome without me realizing it. And when I say a lot of alcohol, it was really a lot so that I got to the point of not being able to drink without vomiting for a few days afterwards.

Secondly, I fell deeply in love with a young man when I was 16 years old in a relationship that lasted until I was 20. When that ended, I was catapulted into a lot of my childhood grief, and instead of feeling that loss and all that it brought up about my childhood, I did everything that I could to not feel, meaning that I drank, and partied and started another relationship with a man who was pretty abusive and intense. All of that avoidance of feeling left me in a high level of stress and tension. In short a lot of grasping.

When you are ignoring the pain, it leaves little option but to push through to make anything happen in your life. The attitude of forcing starts to become a habit.

There was a phase of about five years, on and off, where I catapulted from the conflictual relationship into the high-achieving career, all in a way that was outside of myself. Bouncing out of that deep grief and love for the man who had really touched me to the core sent me into a spin of unconscious disconnection. And in that disconnection there was so much grasping, looking externally for solutions to feel better. Changing my diet, forbidding myself pleasures and then overindulging in those same pleasures until I got sick again. Moving to a new city where I knew no one, changing my whole life. You could say that this was something of an addiction to striving, creating a much repeated pattern of crashing. I was stuck in a yang motion on overdrive. My body had to crash to get any sense of relief and opposite momentum.

When I say that my body had to crash, I experienced it as the only way that I really was able to fully let go and have deep internal peace was when I crashed. In the extreme pain, nausea, debilitating gripping of the collapse, I had to draw the curtains, turn off all electronic devices, come back to my breath, and make it through just one breath at a time. At first, it was excruciating, but as I moved into the intimacy with the intense gripping and the moment-by-moment incremental release, becoming quiet inside, my whole being would begin to let go. That was how I learned to recover, first from the acute grasp of the collapses and then from the whole condition, step by step, learning to release that immense tension in overdrive.

In contrast with the clutching intensity that led me to crash, the ability to sit down and cry, feel deeply, and let go could be seen as part of the yin polarity. As someone who feels very deeply and intensely but learned to hold it all in and just "soldier on," it took about six years of being stuck in overdrive before I was able to find an IST practitioner and utilize IST to be held and let go into the flow of those feelings so that they could be truly released. That was my first awareness of a real yin-doing in my life.

For me, the experience of CFS was at least partly about learning to find harmony between the yin and the yang forces inside of myself, but also to find what Sagan calls "the higher mode."

Both the more watery yin feminine and the more fiery masculine aspects of our energy and consciousness can operate from a lower mode or a higher mode.

The lower mode of the feminine is potentially pleasure-orientated, sleepy and so deeply yin that we will never wake up, and the masculine so driven and grasping that we end up outside of ourselves, in pain and unable to move forward.

There is also a higher mode of the feminine like the ocean, a great power that also carries immense wisdom and inner knowing of the mysteries of the creation. The masculine forces within us can be expressed through a high principle of fire that can bring clarity, motivation, enthusiasm, and awakening.

Even though I was in overdrive on the yang mode, getting better was not as simple as dialing that down, or even creating a sense of balance in yinyang energy. Balance is a good concept and does help, but full recovery was also about turning the polarities to their higher mode. Meaning that the fire of the masculine drive could become more refined and lighter, less graspy, and the yin flowing feminine force within me could be actively receptive, instead of sleepy and depressed.

Don't worry. I will go further into these higher modes, because it is crucial not just for your recovery but really for all of us to reach our higher potential, if that is what we want.

KNOWING THE YINYANG FLOW WITHIN

In my experience many people with CFS or burnout-type of conditions have an inner conflict with their feminine or yin side. If we move through our lives either primarily yin or predominantly yang, we are potentially out of balance. A culture that prioritizes the goal- and action-orientated way of existing and dismisses the more yin power of providing the container, the devotion, the receptive does not encourage people to have harmony.

When I was a financial journalist in the wire industry, life was go, go, go. People that I meet now who are in the media are even more driven by the need to constantly perform, never getting offline even in their downtime.

Taking time out is not a luxury. It is a necessity, not just on holidays but on a daily basis. The pressures of the digital age, social media, and an ever-shifting job market mean that people struggle to switch off at all.

For example, during the 2020 COVID pandemic, there was a time when I was managing a team. I knew things were getting out of balance when I would wake up in the middle of the night to check my texts, stressing out about management decisions and other people's welfare even in my dreams. Like many, many others in the world during that phase, my life was blowing up and imploding at the same time. I could not rest by taking time off. I had to totally break the cycle by leaving that job to get my own peace of mind back and regain some of my ability to rest properly.

When someone is out of balance, it can show up in a lot of tension, emotional chaos, or just physical symptoms that cause real illness. The term *grasping* really does speak to this experience of tension, stress, gripping, and pulling inside. Grasping is a result of the disharmony between the feminine and masculine forces inside of us. This same grasping blocks the healing and regeneration that we really need and is innate in our own bodies.

The dance between feminine and masculine is supposed to move through us throughout the day, and when it cannot flow like this, we get blocked, stuck, and sometimes sick.

The flow is easy to see if you look back at the energy of the day. The rising fire of sunrise, the creative action of the morning, the high time of connection with each other and the world at noon, and late afternoon, the drowsy time when a desire to nap or just rest quietly pulls at us. Later, there is more yang time as the afternoon moves on, a mode of getting things done and preparing for the next day, before we return to the great yin in the hour of dusk, where our consciousness rests in between day and night, grasping neither but somehow present in both.

These rhythms are not necessarily personal. They exist all around us and inside of our bodies. But we start to disconnect from ourselves when we fight them with caffeine, pushing ourselves, striving, and driving for more and more productivity and achievement. In effect, we negate the yin movements when our body of energy yearns for quiet introspection and reflection. There is also no real room for that sense of inner peace that comes with the ability to become more internalized, more yin in ourselves.

I have been extremely action-orientated and goal-focused for much of my life, but when that started to override my actual need for rest, for sleep, for contemplation, for healing, for feeling and letting go of my grief, I crashed. The pushing, forcing, driving energy became so strong that my life force was completely depleted, and it collapsed. This was not a minor collapse as in a bad hangover that takes a few days to recover from. It was a major collapse that continued to create havoc in my body for years until I changed my life completely.

I am not alone in this. Many people with CFS, burnout, post-viral fatigue, or even Lyme disease who I have interviewed or worked with as a practitioner were living their lives at a pace that was unsustainable when they first got sick. Whether that was with work, with partying, or just plain old being intensely out of balance. And it took many of them a long time to address this imbalance because it is so deeply ingrained in our collective psyche.

MORE AWARENESS OF FLOW INSTEAD OF SLOWING DOWN

Living at a slower pace won't necessarily make people better. Rather, we need to be able to monitor where we are at and when we need to shift from creative to receptive as needed, so that we know how to avert a crash. This happens on a moment-to-moment basis and comes from a deep sense of connection to our own core.

Our bodies and the force of life within us are part of this feminine principle. Yet we do not know how to look after our energy, our physical bodies, nor be connected at this level.

Processed food, takeout, and a lot more meat and junk than the body can take in makes us sick. We do less exercise than our bodies need and get less sleep than our bodies need for the most part. All of these things cause major physical health issues, yet they are a symptom of the disconnection that is happening in the whole world.

This imbalance is something that plagues all of humanity at the moment. The resulting disconnection inside of ourselves shows up in our relationship to nature, which is the feminine or yin. As we all know, human beings are ruining the planet with pollution, climate change, unsustainable farming practices, and simple lack of respect. Most of the human inhabitants of this Earth see nature as separate to us, and therefore the issues which we know are deeply pressing and have been for a long time now, seem to be largely irrelevant to our daily lives.

We are becoming increasingly caught up in our heads, stimulated by the world around us and rapidly changing technology. This cuts us off from being able to feel and know what our bodies (and the nature that our bodies are inherently part of) need.

CASE STUDY – MICHELLE TAPPING INTO THE FLOW OF SENSUALITY

Michelle in Toronto, Canada was about 52 years old and had suffered CFS for about 22 years when I first saw her as a client for IST.

She initially had some bad injuries on horses and in yoga classes that resulted in a lot of chronic back and neck pain. Then she became increasingly fatigued, weighed down with brain fog, and started crashing intensely when she was in her late 20s. It never really got any better. Sometimes she spent weeks in bed, and at other times she was dragging herself through studies and a career as a psychiatrist.

In terms of her yinyang flow, she was stuck in a chronic level of pain and grasping, unable to let go and have any kind of relief or energetic sense of receptivity at all.

She was a tall willowy blonde who had what I would call extremely feminine energy, but when I first met her, she was out of touch with it and uncomfortable with it. Her long thin body seemed almost twisted in a tight gripping pain. Her body was often locked in a posture of tension and discomfort.

When she laughed, her whole face would light up with joy, and her demeanor opened like a shining sun. Most of the time, though, she was brooding and unhappy, nursing some kind of pain or fatigue, fighting herself on the inside.

One thing about Michelle that was surprising was that even though she was pretty conservative in her life and her presentation, when we did IST, she had an incredibly vibrant yin-flowing energy in her lower centers.

People are not the same in their body of energy. We are all quite different. Michelle was unusual for someone of her demeanor because her energy below was full of beauty and life and vibrancy. Almost like it was singing in colors and vibrations. She shared that when we went inside to feel those lower aspects of her body of energy, it was also highly sensual and even sexual in her experience. Yet she lived most of her life completely and painfully cut off from that flowing force inside.

Michelle felt challenged because she was married to a man with whom she had absolutely no sexual connection at all. She loved him, and they cared for each other deeply, but they did not have any sexual chemistry, she said. They had been married for 12 years, and in that time had very little (if any) satisfying sex. But she did not want to leave him even though she felt it was tying her belly up in knots. He took care of her in different ways; she was scared to be alone.

Michelle was a good example of someone who was in conflict with her own yinyang knowhow.

We all have feminine and masculine energy within us. We have both polarities all of the time. Some people tend to experience one polarity more than the other, but they are both there inside of us. And they flow through every single day and the whole of life.

In her life, Michelle spent a lot of her time in fear, even terror, trying to avoid the days of pain that crashing brought in its wake. She controlled her diet and often reacted to her husband because he wasn't able to help her in the way that she thought she needed. And who could blame her? She was suffering a lot.

After so many years of CFS, Michelle was also one of those people who was sometimes very difficult to be around because she was prickly and extremely picky, complaining and having the unintentional effect of pulling down the space around her. Her pain was excruciating at times, and this was broadcast in her behavior.

Meanwhile, her husband looked beaten down, lugging all the supplements, foods, special cushions, or whatever she needed around to whichever workshops she would attend in the hope of getting better.

Like many people that I have seen with CFS and other fatigue and pain-related illnesses, including fibromyalgia, Michelle was often gripped in pain and related to the term *grasping* experientially.

"I get stuck in this grasping, and it kind of turns in on itself until I collapse with a migraine, and unbearable pain," she said when seeing me for a round of IST sessions. "The grasping is so great that I am often unable to make it let go, no matter what I do. Sometimes just lying in a dark room with complete quiet for a few days makes it all let go, and I am released until the next one comes along. But stepping outside of it when it first starts seems impossible." Michelle winced as she talked and shook her head.

When we explored this grasping mechanism within the sessions, it turned out that a few years previously, when Michelle had been seeing the male healer whom she fell in love with at the time, there was a phase of over a year where she was totally without pain and grasping. In fact she was in bliss.

It seemed to her at the time that the healer was giving her a sensual awakening. She called it a "kundalini awakening." But she felt as if he did it to her. Alongside that, she did what many others would do too in this situation. She fell in love with that healer. After a kind of twisted turn of events where it looked like they would have an affair, he told her that he did not requite her feelings. This turned into another reason to twist against herself rather than offering a long-term cure.

In this case, Michelle's power and her sexual energy were entwined. As a result of her upbringing, she had some deep-held beliefs that she could not be in this part of herself. And yet there it was, in the first session that we did together, available almost immediately. It was almost as if she was waiting for someone else to give her permission to be that alive.

This was where we saw Michelle's "stubborn resistance." Her feminine and irrational nature would not give up on the healer being the answer to her problems, even though her mind had decided it was impossible, especially given that after a little while of flirtations and sensual connection, the healer deliberately broke away from her, asking her to go elsewhere for her treatments. At that point Michelle was catapulted back into her misery, physical and emotional. All of her CFS symptoms returned, and the state of bliss that she was in while there was a connection with her healer was all gone.

It is difficult when something like this happens because it is not clear what is right and what is wrong. If it had been possible, should Michelle have left her husband and explored the affair with this man who gave her a sense of bliss and freedom? There was a point where she really contemplated it. Or should she have stayed with the reliability of her marriage and best friend even though her sexual self was in misery and she was blocked and in pain?

Regardless of whether she should or could have left her husband or whether she could have opened up a more satisfying connection with him, Michelle did use the IST sessions to get in touch with that sensual aspect of herself and start to choose it inside of herself instead of pushing it away.

Many times when we explore the deeper parts of ourselves, it is not just the trauma and the old wounds that we have kept inside, nor just the things we consider to be bad like our violence or rage, but also the good things, our superpowers that we have kept hidden even from ourselves.

Michelle was someone who had hidden this powerful sensual vitality that she had from herself. It was something that her mother had reacted strongly against, and although she was not conscious of it as a child, she had turned it in on itself in order to stay in favor.

Clearing that cage-like relationship with her mother and her own sexuality gave Michelle a sense of her power separate from anyone or anything else. It gave her freedom to be in her own sense of pleasure and shift toward a life that was not continually reinforcing that cage. Her CFS symptoms shifted significantly when she broke up with her husband, and allowed herself to explore her sexuality even though she had judged herself too old at the age of 50.

Using the meditation-based techniques for inner exploration in our sessions together, Michelle was also able to learn to ignite her own life force energy below. Through first using the interactive sessions to learn the pathway to experiencing and engaging those energies, and later learning to follow the pathway of awakening herself in silent meditation practice on a daily basis, Michelle was able to ignite that power below.

The sessions were about Michelle learning to step into that flowing, feminine sense of visceral pleasure in her body at will. The male healer had given her a taste of something, but the IST needed to show her that this bliss was inside of herself and available to her all of the time, not something that someone else would give her permission to feel.

The body of life force is a body of sexual energy. Life is about reproduction. When our vitality is turned on, there is highly likely going to be more access to sexual pleasure and wellbeing. When Michelle felt sexy, she often felt a lot more vital and well than when she was actively and unconsciously shutting that part of herself down.

Michelle is not alone finding relief from her pain through accessing her sexual energy, as studies have shown that many people with a history of migraines and cluster headaches for example do find relief through sexual pleasure.

A 2013 study from the University of Munster in Germany, resulting from a survey distributed to 1,000 patients diagnosed with either migraines or cluster headaches found:

- Around 60 percent of people with migraines reported an improvement of their headaches with sexual activity.
- Of the people with migraines who found improvement in their headaches with sexual activity, over one-third of the males and almost 14 percent of the females used sexual activity as a regular therapeutic tool.
- About 43 percent of people with migraines found that their headache changed shortly after orgasm or maximal excitement, almost 18 percent reported the change with the time of orgasm, 20 percent found the change at the beginning of sexual activity while another 20 percent had the change within 30 minutes of orgasm or maximal excitement. This change did not depend on type of sexual activity, partner, time of the migraine attack, or position during sex.[39]

The report on the Association of Migraine Disorders website, medically reviewed by Dr. Megan Donnelly, says that:

- Interestingly, orgasm and pain affect some of the same areas of the brain, including the cortex, hypothalamus and more.

---

39. Stefan Evers et al., "Prevalence of Cluster Headache in Germany: Results of the Epidemiological DMKG Study," *Journal of Neurology, Neurosurgery, and Psychiatry*, November 2007, https://www.ncbi.nlm.nih.gov/pmc/articles/PMC2117619.

- Orgasms stimulate the production of endorphins, marvelous neurochemicals released from the brain that act like opioids, providing rapid pain relief that is even stronger than morphine! To put it in a simple equation: sexual orgasm=endorphin production=pain relief or analgesia.
- During a migraine attack, people may have lower levels of certain neurotransmitters like dopamine and serotonin. Both of these neurotransmitters are released during sexual activity.
- Sex may also be beneficial for migraine because it distracts a person from the pain.[40]

For Michelle at times it might have been about having sex or orgasms, but really it was about being connected to her own body in a sensual and pleasure-orientated way on a daily basis. This experience was not just physical but energetic. Enjoying the way she moved, feeling the pleasure in her food, her garden, her bathing, anything that made her body of energy happy on a moment-to-moment basis. Choosing this more yin or receptive motion inside of herself instead of the motion of grasping and retraction that had built up years and years of pain.

---

40. Lisa Smith, "Everything You Wanted to Know about Sex and Migraines (but Were Afraid to Ask!)," Association of Migraine Disorders, February 23, 2024, https://www.migrainedisorders.org/everything-you-wanted-to-know-about-sex-and-migraines-but-were-afraid-to-ask/.

She wasn't able to access that before the IST sessions, except with the healer's help. Through the IST sessions, she was able to go deeper inside to find a connection with those feeling parts inside of herself, allowing them to be irrational, getting to know their irrepressible and mysterious nature, finding a way to navigate that allowed both the rational mind and the deeper more subtle feminine self to coexist instead of fighting each other all of the time.

Oftentimes, people with this kind of CFS or burnout have some kind of twisted relationship to their own energy of desire or wanting. It turns in on itself and therefore drains their vitality enormously. I know this was the case for myself, but I also observed it in many clients and case histories that I have gathered over the last 20 years.

I have found that working with people to help them get into the depths of vitality and aliveness in their own lower centers of energy is often a pretty fast way to create a pathway for a positive health shift.

Many clients who have come to see me with CFS-type of issues have had huge forces of life in their energy centers below that they are in fact twisted against or shutting themselves away from unconsciously. The clients do not realize that they have turned away from this huge resource in their own body of energy. In many cases, it does not take a lot to help the client to see their own massive forces of life available below.

People have different strengths and weaknesses, varying talents and abilities in their subtle bodies just as they do in their physical bodies. Some folks really have vital and glowing life force energy that gives them a vibrancy. For example, some people who are famous actors have such glowing and vital life force energy that it is magnetic, attracting a lot of attention and admiration.

I do not have a why, but many people with the CFS-type of profile who have come to me for support have what I would call a big energy in the centers below, and when they can see this and consciously tap into it, they do experience a major boost in their health.

I was one of those with a big voltage of life below who had unconsciously shut down the vibrancy of that force in myself, probably to do with my own voracious sexuality since a very young age. I shut it down to be acceptable, because of various unrequited love affairs, and family and social conditioning.

Opening myself to experience the joy, the vitality, the sensuality of those energies for no reason except to appreciate myself was a big part of the mid-phase of my recovery.

7

TECHNOLOGY & THE MODERN AGE CONTRIBUTING TO THE FATIGUE EPIDEMIC

At all stages of recovering from CFS and burnout types of illness, managing the impact of technology and the modern world is key. Particularly as so many people now, even those without CFS/ME or burnout, have experiences of crashing when they are hauled up online for too long.

I remember noticing communities of people living off the grid in both Western Australia and northern New South Wales were still under stress, angry, burdened by the intense emotions and demands of the modern world.

Like it or not, we are living in the technological age where the extreme fast pace of change keeps us moving at breakneck speeds. Without self-awareness, this potential mayhem can propel us further and further into a depleted unhealthy and lower masculine type of pushing.

Even if we step away from the technology itself, and go off the grid, human consciousness has changed over the time as our world has shifted. People's emotions are faster, bigger, more intense. We are operating at a different level of astral energy than was even available prior to World War 1.

The global shift in technology is clearly impacting our minds, as well as our vitality and wellbeing on a deeper level.

"Never before have a handful of tech designers had such control over the way billions of us think, act, and live our lives," says the documentary *The Social Dilemma*.[41]

There is a movement to align technology with humanity's best interest, created by Tristan Harris after his presentation "A Call to Minimize Distraction & Respect Users' Attention" went viral in 2013 when he was a Google Design Ethicist. Along with partners, Harris set up the Center for Humane Technology (CHT) envisioning "a world with technology that respects our attention, improves our wellbeing, and strengthens communities."[42]

---

41. *The Social Dilemma*, March 14, 2022, Netflix, https://www.thesocialdilemma.com/.

42. "About Us," Center for Humane Technology, accessed July 8, 2024, https://www.humanetech.com/who-we-are.

In 2017, a 5,000 person study found that higher social media use correlated with self-reported declines in mental and physical health and life satisfaction.[43]

In 2021 an article in the Guardian reported that *"Researchers have long complained that little is shared publicly regarding how, exactly, Facebook algorithms work, what is being shared privately on the platform, and what information Facebook collects on users."* Kari Paul went on to add in the article that, "Facebook's own researchers found that '64% of all extremist group joins are due to our recommendation tools,' an internal report in 2016 found."[44]

Frances Haugen, a former product manager at Facebook, testified in 2021 in front of the Senate on the impact of the company on society. Haugan said that she came forward after she saw Facebook's leadership repeatedly prioritize profit over safety, according to an article in the *MIT Technology Review*. Social media on the whole can be seen in the light that Haugen shines on Facebook. She said in her opening statement to lawmakers,

---

43. Holly B. Shakya and Nicholas A. Christakis, "Association of Facebook Use with Compromised Well-Being: A Longitudinal Study," *American Journal of Epidemiology* 185, no. 3 (January 16, 2017): 203–11, https://doi.org/10.1093/aje/kww189.

44. Kari Paul, "'It Let White Supremacists Organize': The Toxic Legacy of Facebook's Groups," *The Guardian*, February 4, 2021, https://www.theguardian.com/technology/2021/feb/04/facebook-groups-misinformation.

I'm here today because I believe Facebook's products harm children, stoke division, and weaken our democracy... These problems are solvable. A safer, free-speech respecting, more enjoyable social media is possible. But there is one thing that I hope everyone takes away from these disclosures—it is that Facebook can change, but is clearly not going to do so on its own.[45]

Alongside all of these really important points regarding the impact of technology on human consciousness, I would like to add that it potentially has a significant impact on our life force or vital energies.

Have you ever been working at full tilt for such a long period of time that when you do attempt to stop and take your foot off of the accelerator, you lie down and just cannot rest? At some point you have to get up and do something even though you are totally and utterly exhausted because the mind just will not stop?

It is almost impossible in those states to shift gears into a yin-type release. For me when I am in that overdrive, I know I wake up in the middle of the night with hectic dreams that I am late for an important meeting. I'll even sleepwalk to solve some illusory crisis.

---

45. Karen Hao, "The Facebook Whistleblower Says Its Algorithms Are Dangerous. Here's Why.," *MIT Technology Review*, June 29, 2022, https://www.technologyreview.com/2021/10/05/1036519/facebook-whistleblower-frances-haugen-algorithms/.

This kind of on-switch that won't turn off is a sign that burnout or some kind of collapse looms, and usually is the result of pushing beyond the physical and subtle bodies' capacity.

Interestingly, if you have not yet crashed, but are just totally buzzed out, sometimes getting up and doing physical exercise that makes you sweat, especially if it is outside in nature, will bring the body back to a good kind of collapse where you can sleep and let go. It was the overexertion of the mind, not the physical body, that caused the wired state of sleeplessness.

But if you have CFS or Long COVID or even some types of burnout, any kind of exercise can leave you unwell or bedridden for days. That is called post-exertion malaise (PEM).

Essentially, those more fiery, yang, pushing mechanisms can go so far into overdrive that nothing seems to work to bring the body back to equilibrium and rest. When the overexertion has been pushed so far that there is really no juice left in the life force, or etheric body, even bedrest for days and days does not result in wellness or relief. This could be because that pushing has resulted in some kind of major crash that needs addressing at the level of subtle bodies.

This on-switch in overdrive that left us exhausted happened because at some point we forgot how to listen to our bodies and knowing. We lost the ability to turn inside, to be reflective, to receive the wisdom from within. That is when the crashing became inevitable.

EXTREME FATIGUE, CRASHING OR COLLAPSING OF VITALITY AND SUBTLE BODIES

Samuel Sagan predicted that there will be a marked increase in CFS-related health disorders, including something that he termed Chronic Fatigue Psychosis.

The logical outcome of subtle body trends that are already solidly established. The 21st century will see a very dramatic increase in CFS-related health disorders. For some patients, Chronic Fatigue will become so bad that it will border on psychosis. Sufferers will lie in bed with vacant eyes, as if gone.

CFS, or CFP, Chronic Fatigue Psychosis, will take on the proportions of an epidemic. Large numbers of people will be put totally out of action, which could put significant stress on the resources of the community.

This is not unavoidable. There are ways to prevent this disaster. But a real solution cannot come from yet another brilliant discovery by pharmaceutical companies. It is not a drug that can resolve this problem, but an action where the source of the problem really lies—in the balance of subtle bodies.[46]

The current environment that we are in now is creating conditions for increased chronic fatigue-type symptoms including the chronic psychosis type of conditions that Sagan referred to above.

There is increasing astral stimulation from the growing intensity of our political, corporate, and online environments. And the amount of time that people spend on technology including their cell phones, online conferences, and video games has gone up exponentially.

FATIGUE IS ALREADY AT EPIDEMIC PROPORTIONS AROUND THE GLOBE

We have a world where many people are suffering from intense and long-standing fatigue, including CFS, Long COVID, and the increasing occurrence of debilitating cases of burnout.

From a standpoint of understanding subtle bodies, some of those people with burnout or ongoing unexplained fatigue are experiencing severe crashing in their vital energy. To say

---

46. Samuel Sagan MD, *KT FuXi's Mountain*, Point Horizon Institute. 2011, written PDF for an online correspondence course, *293*. Quote used with the kind permission of Samuel Sagan, 2008.

that someone is crashing does not disregard the presence of physical issues, but resolving the energetic component can make the physical issues far easier to address.

These illnesses probably have more than one root cause, but the symptoms of intense and completely debilitating fatigue are something that they have in common. As I said at the beginning, CFS is a kind of umbrella term coined by the CDC and the World Health Organization (WHO) in the 1990s for a group of symptoms that at the time had no known cause.

In my experience the crossover between CFS, burnout, and even Long COVID is that people in all of those categories can be suffering from a profound crash or collapse in their subtle bodies. Not everyone who has CFS, burnout, or Long COVID has had such a crash, but those who are in this category may be missing out on looking at their subtle bodies and vital life force energy for a real cure or transition back to full health.

This is such an important part of the puzzle because the occurrence of people crashing or collapsing is fast increasing, affecting their ability to contribute to their families, their communities, and even their jobs in any meaningful way.

A crash, described in the earlier chapters, is when the energy of thoughts and emotions floods the subtle life force causing many intense symptoms including physical pain, migraines, brain fog, sleep issues, digestion or gut issues, and sometimes the inability to get out of bed for days, weeks, or months.

Burnout, CFS, and Long COVID are different illnesses, but they all end up with this absolutely debilitating, even crushing fatigue, along with an array of other symptoms that vary from one person to the next. These include fatigue, brain fog, post-exertion malaise, headaches and migraines, digestive issues, and even increased allergies and sensitivities.

It is not that they are all the same thing, but that there is some crossover at a cultural and individual level when it comes to the underlying issue in terms of subtle bodies. We push our life force or etheric bodies too far over the line and keep using the astral stimulants to the point that we are completely over-taxed.

There are a number of studies that point to the link between increased astral energy (the energy of emotions and thoughts) and fatigue.[47]

Sagan was highlighting that as the world becomes more and more intense, and people's thoughts and emotions are increasingly potent or weighty, he saw more and more people having what he called Chronic Fatigue Psychosis.

---

47. S. B. Harvey et al., "The Relationship between Prior Psychiatric Disorder and Chronic Fatigue: Evidence from a National Birth Cohort Study," Psychological Medicine 38, no. 7 (November 2, 2007): 933–40, https://doi.org/10.1017/s0033291707001900.

BURNING THE FLAME, YINYANG IMBALANCE GONE VIRAL

Whether the intense grasping of consciousness causes emotional or physical pain or both, it is the antipathy of flow.

In a healthy human experience using the model of yinyang flow, these two poles are meant to oscillate throughout our day and our lives. We spend time in nature; we go to the city. We sleep and let go at night; we enter our full state of engagement during the day. Like a flow of yinyang, engaging and pressing in, then flowing back to letting go and regeneration.

Unfortunately, there is no letting go when you are always plugged in. Here astral consciousness is overbearing or gripping and draining the pole of life or the etheric. When people are constantly plugged in, their senses are being triggered all day, pulling them out of their own grounded sense of center, and also draining their vitality. The astral body is always gripping the etheric, or life principle. There is no room for regeneration.

Seeing the whole problem at the level of subtle bodies can bring another dimension to the issue, and help us to gain more clarity about what is happening here.

In my experience with clients with burnout, some people in this category are also crashing intensely. A good night of sleep, a weekend off, or even a week off does not regenerate or refresh someone in this state. It takes a long time to recover, and often that recovery involves a total reevaluation of their lifestyle and how that person chooses to engage their energy on a daily basis.

People who are crashing like this can experience symptoms like very bad headaches, migraines, ongoing flu-like symptoms, exhaustion, and other CFS-like symptoms. Others are more emotionally stressed and drained.

In terms of understanding subtle bodies, this results in a very high level of emotional and intellectual stimulation that never lets up, meaning that the pole of consciousness or astral energies outweighs the pole of life or etheric.

It is like being stuck in an out-of-balance yinyang flow, always in action, never being able to let go and drop into the more feminine state in order to be receptive, introspective, quiet, and internal.

HOW TECHNOLOGY IMPACTS VITALITY AND LEADS TO BURNOUT

Technology stimulates the astral body or our consciousness, potentially creating non-stop grasping of the etheric or body of life force. It is immensely draining if we never get to really let go. I am not advocating getting rid of technology here, but a healthy assessment of boundaries with our gadgets. As we are increasingly plugged in almost 24/7, we hardly ever get to switch off.

Essentially, burnout happens when people are in unhealthy, highly stimulating work environments that end up causing deep levels of fatigue. And burnout is more likely to happen when people are feeling conflicted in themselves with the underlying reason they are doing that job in the first place. Much like I felt as a financial journalist, many who end with burnout do not feel connected to a real sense of "why do this job?"

As a finance journalist in wire, I had three screens on my desk and two phones. I would flip from screen to screen, doing several things at once. And by the time that I was in the peak of that career, I was fast, very fast. I did all of the work that was required of me and more, often writing up to 5,000 words a day, resulting in phases when story after story was published day after day in newspapers around the country.

It was so exciting to rush to the papers and flick through to the finance section to see where our stories were published, cutting them out to make our scrapbooks. It gave me a rush to do things fast, to make the news and put out minute-by-minute headlines. I felt big and powerful when I walked into press conferences along with the other journalists from different media outlets, and asked the CEO and the PR people hard-hitting questions.

Yet I was never really into finance or markets or corporate news at all. Prior to becoming a journalist, I was an activist, campaigning to save forests and whales, and had been a vegetarian for a lot of my life. So once I got the big wins, and was really beginning to fly in that career, the shine wore off. I started to feel and see the emptiness and the lack of warmth in that industry. I felt deeply conflicted.

Then I got sick, a bad infection on my left foot after it was cut on a broken mirror. Some strong antibiotics. A severe flu that I did not give enough time to heal. Always rushing back to work before my body was ready. Forcing and pushing myself to show up and be more. Yet in the background, I yearned for something else, and I did not even know what that something else would be.

During this time, the phones were buzzing, the alarm went off before the sun rose, there were regular trips to the coffee shop to keep myself awake, and a lot of constant stimulation and intense stress.

I hit that point where stress flips from being stimulating and alive, driving me forward and keeping me on my toes, to being something that's exhausting, even deeply depleting.

Very quickly, I could no longer drink a couple of beers with colleagues after work without being sick—really, really sick, all day the next day. The food that I ate began to slide through me the minute that I ingested it.

In a matter of weeks, it seemed like sleep began to take on new proportions, dragging me into its clutches like a heavy sandman so that I felt like I would never come back. Over the next few months, my body started to be heavy and painful all of the time, and even mild exercise began to give me a lot more pain and fatigue than it ever had before.

I started to have incredibly painful migraines for the first time in my life, even vomiting with the pain. But nothing gave me relief except lying in a cool dark room until it went away.

But still I pushed and pushed, forcing myself to keep going, to keep fighting, to keep striving to win.

The high level of stimulation in an active wire news room has a buzz a bit like a war office. The deadlines are constant, minute by minute, second by second. Everyone's working faster than they're physically capable of and doing it for longer hours than their bodies can actually withstand over days and weeks and months and years.

When I was working in the news-wire, the deputy finance news editor had a debilitatingly painful back injury; the finance editor got pneumonia and seemed unable to recover for months and months. We all watched him struggling on at his desk as soon as he was out of hospital and could get up. Everyone on the finance floor seemed to be looking for another job at one point because they felt fried and exhausted.

From where I sat, in the corner desk with a view of the elevator, it looked like this office was a haven of burnout, although I did not really understand what that was at the time. I just saw people working really hard and getting ill.

We weren't alone here. People in the stock exchange, at the fund managers, in the big investment firms, at the law firms, in the major hospitals, also commonly burned out. And as the world became more and more hooked up, burnout burgeoned.

For me, burnout was part of my story even though I was diagnosed with CFS.

Based on all the work that I have done over the years in this area, I do see that in some cases there is crossover between burnout and CFS, although they are not the same thing.

Chronic Fatigue is already something of an umbrella term, and sometimes it might be used to describe people with very bad burnout and vice versa. Meaning that a component of people with burnout do crash energetically, and a component of people with CFS do have some history of burnout. I know that I did.

When I was studying CFS and burnout for my master's thesis in the early 2000s, it was obvious to me that some people who were diagnosed with burnout had very similar symptoms to some people who were diagnosed with CFS, although their illnesses might have had very different causes.

In some cases there is a crossover between CFS and burnout. Remember that CFS is something of an umbrella term labeling a set of symptoms without any clear sense of the underlying cause. Sometimes the underlying cause of CFS can be related to burnout or the same as very severe situations of burnout. I will spell out more of this when I talk about CFS and willpower in the coming chapters.

In medical terms, CFS/ME has been linked to viral infections. Additionally, I have seen a number of cases where there were also lifestyle-related causes to the issues at hand for the person with CFS, and resolving those lifestyle issues meant they recovered from CFS and whatever viral infection they had much quicker.

WHY IS FATIGUE PLAGUING THE MODERN WORLD RIGHT NOW?

Fast forward to 2020 and everyone was working at breakneck speed, when COVID-19 hit and we all went into isolation at the same time as the super-fast pace of change in technology started to crest into a world where everyone can be online 10-plus hours a day at home, including 5 to 10 Zoom meetings every day.

That is when the term Zoom fatigue quickly became the new norm.

Zoom fatigue is a new phenomenon illustrating how technology relates to burnout and the fatigue epidemic that we face right now in the world post-COVID.

The Psychiatric Times put out an article on Zoom fatigue in November 2020 saying:

"Zoom fatigue" describes the tiredness, worry, or burnout associated with overusing virtual platforms of communication. Like other experiences associated with the coronavirus (COVID-19) pandemic, Zoom fatigue is widely prevalent, intense, and completely new.[48]

The Zoom mobile app was downloaded **485 million times** in 2020. Compared with the same quarter of the previous year, annual Zoom meeting minutes increased by **3300 percent** in October 2020.[49]

Researchers have said that this new type of fatigue comes from the difference in communication on Zoom and the rapid eye movement. With the increase in working from home in 2020 during COVID, people have also increased the number of online meetings they attend per day up to 5 or even 10 meetings a day. *"Some people have as many as nine or ten video meetings in a day."*[50]

Kate Smith at CBS reported in 2021 that more women have experienced the impact of Zoom fatigue than men: *"Some*

---

48. Jena Lee, "A Neuropsychological Exploration of Zoom Fatigue," *Psychiatric Times*, November 17, 2020, https://www.psychiatrictimes.com/view/psychological-exploration-zoom-fatigue.

49. Brian Dean, "Zoom User Stats: How Many People Use Zoom?," Backlinko, February 13, 2024, https://backlinko.com/zoom-users.

50. Kif Leswing, "Why We're Experiencing 'Zoom Fatigue' and How to Fix It," CNBC, February 25, 2021, https://www.cnbc.com/2021/02/25/zoom-fatigue-why-we-have-it-how-to-fix-it.html.

are reporting headaches, feeling drained, and loss of enthusiasm regarding their work and colleagues. Researchers have shown more women are impacted than men."[51]

From my standpoint as an IST practitioner and former finance journalist, people have been experiencing these symptoms relating to deep immersion in all sorts of technology for the last 20 years. But of course it has become much more common and increasingly intense as a result of the huge increase in working from home that happened in 2020 and the resulting fact that technology then gained even more traction in our lives.

And it is easy to see that it will become even more prevalent. Mustafa Suleyman in his book *The Coming Wave* makes it clear that we are only a few years away from AI becoming "inextricably part of the social fabric."[52]

> *...Our brains are terrible at making sense of the rapid scaling of an exponential, and so in a field like AI it's not always easy to grasp what is actually happening. It's inevitable that in the next years and decades many orders of magnitude more compute will be used to train*

---

51. Kate Smith, "Women Experience Higher Levels of 'Zoom Fatigue' than Men, Study Finds," CBS News, April 21, 2021, https://www.cbsnews.com/news/zoom-fatigue-women-higher-men/.

52. Mustafa Suleyman and Michael Bhaskar, *The Coming Wave: AI, Power and the Twenty-First Century's Greatest Dilemma* (London: Jonathan Cape, 2023), 61.

the largest AI models, and so, if the scaling hypothesis is at least partially true, there is an inevitability about what this means.[53]

Suleyman also points to the way that the current technological advancements will result in a huge shift in what human beings become. The convergence of biology and engineering, like AI and synthetic biology, sends us on a trajectory to a new kind of human.

...At the center of this wave sits the realization that DNA is information, a biologically evolved encoding and storage system. Over recent decades we have come to understand enough about this information transmission system that we can now intervene to alter its encoding and direct its course. As a result, food, medicine, materials, manufacturing processes and consumer goods will all be transformed and re-imagined. So will humans themselves.[54]

In terms of subtle bodies, firstly there is a huge leap in the amount of mental stimulation the more time that we spend online, and particularly with more video or even virtual reality.

But then, as we start to play with biology and life itself, there is another dice thrown with our relationship to this

---

53. Mustafa Suleyman, *The Coming Wave*, 67.

54. Mustafa Suleyman, *The Coming Wave*, 79.

vital element of our subtle bodies. The connection between the mind or consciousness and life itself potentially begins to split further and further apart.

We already have something of a divorce between consciousness or the astral body and life or the etheric that creates a detrimental imbalance in our subtle bodies.

As the mind is stimulated with lights, sounds, and frequencies of consciousness that do not relate to where we are actually sitting with our physical bodies, our mental energy goes up. You could say that there is more astral stimulation with the increased voltage, buzz, excitement or emotional response required. Every time a text comes through or a social media notification pings, there is a response in the astral body. This leaves our life force under constant attack.

As the energy of our astrality or consciousness is increasingly stimulated and the etheric or life force depleted, the conditions for crashing are ripe.

This imbalance can be addressed, possibly even into the future developments of biotechnology, if we take care of these aspects of our own core nature. Awareness of the lack of balance between the astral and etheric energies within ourselves will go a long way towards giving us the knowledge to adjust and recreate balance. But on its own the etheric or vital energy of our bodies has just not adapted to the new environment. The body of life force is like a very sophisticated nonphysical muscle that needs to work out every day, but is ideally stimulated at its own level with exercise, time in nature, physical contact with our loved ones, and so on.

I am not advocating a return to nature and shift away from technology, or that anyone should slow down their lives. Withdrawing from the world does not change the fact that there is an imbalance even though it can help temporarily if you have crashed. In my experience, total withdrawal from this modern life can make chronic exhaustion much worse.

Selective unplugging, creating better boundaries with technology, even phases of total detox can be very powerful. But a total retraction without any discernment can make someone collapse even more intensely. At least it did for me and a few others that I have worked with in recent years.

We just need to be smarter and more aware of how we are interacting with our tech gadgets, so that they can be developed and utilized in a way that is supportive of our subtle body development instead of making us sick.

"Containment" is the word that people like Tristan Harris and Mustafa Suleyman have been using, indicating that we put boundaries on the onslaught of change, with foresight and awareness of what it is doing and where it is going, making decisions to shape which way it goes rather than trying to stop the momentum that is already well and truly here.

CASE STUDY - JONATHON WITH BURNOUT AND CFS AT AGE 25

Jonathon had CFS as a medical diagnosis, after driving himself extremely hard in his studies and crashing badly. He could have easily been diagnosed with burnout as well because he was in a state of intense overwhelm around his work. He was online and burning the candle at both ends using technology, at the same time as experiencing emotional overload with a very challenging family situation in the background of his life.

He was 25 years old when he came to see me in New York City for some IST sessions. While suffering from extreme fatigue, he had managed to complete a degree in physics and engineering at an Ivy League school on the East Coast of the US. He was intellectually brilliant but really struggled emotionally and physically in his life. He had so many things he wanted to do but could hardly get out of bed for more than a few hours a day.

At the time Jonathon's father was dying of Multiple Sclerosis (MS), which was creating a very heavy dark cloud over his life. As a coping mechanism, Jonathon was spending all of his time online working on his studies and side projects, burying himself in his love for technology. He didn't realize it, but he was frying his etheric through his avid passion for technology, and at the same time, this driven relationship to his work was partially a way of avoiding the awful feelings he had about his connection with his father.

He explained with a scowl that his dad had been very angry ever since he got the diagnosis just over 20 years prior. His father had taken all of the family money to finance treatment for his expensive illness, creating bitter family battles that had dragged out since Jonathon was three years old. There was a lot of resentment and unspoken anger among his siblings and his mother because of the way that his father had behaved. But the illness was so awful, and no one wanted to confront his father so they ended up pushing down all of that emotional toxicity, pretending that it did not exist. It was exhausting for the whole family and a major contributor to Jonathon's illness.

The IST sessions brought Jonathon to the bitterness, rage, and hurt that he had carried in his body from his own sense of abandonment and outrage about his father, but also that he had taken on from his father and mother. Jonathon was carrying not only his own emotions in his body but also the toxic emotions of his father. It was more than a psychological connection. There was an energetic connection, something like a cord of energy, or a deep imprint of the energy of the baggage between the two men.

The IST sessions were as much about helping Jonathon to separate out from his dad's projection of the toxic emotion and energy, as facilitating the release of his own suppressed burdensome feelings regarding the situation. He felt it as a deep betrayal that his dad had never been able to be supportive or kind or holding for him and his siblings during their childhood. Now his dad was dying, and the emotional/energetic sickness around the situation was really impacting Jonathon's health. He himself was almost crippled.

It was really important for Jonathon to get into the visceral experience of expressing the pent-up emotions and feelings about his dad because that energy was keeping him very stuck. So much rage, betrayal, confusion, hurt was dragging him down. It needed to be released.

Releasing his own suppressed emotions about the situation was not enough to make him better, though. There was a toxic, heavy energetic connection between him and his father. This energetic cord or tie between them that was literally sucking on Jonathon's life force.

As a result Jonathon was dragging himself to studies and his many side projects, but sleeping 10 hours to 18 hours at a stretch without a sense of relief or being refreshed at all. He spent most of his waking hours online because he was working on projects that would later be groundbreaking in both gaming and cryptocurrency industries.

In the sessions we went through the major events in Jonathon's life when he had taken on his dad's very heavy emotional and physical burden. Being the oldest son, there was an unconscious expectation that he be responsible for everyone involved, as if from the early age of three he had become the man of the family even though his dad was still alive.

As we separated out those energies, event by event, Jonathon's own vitality started to return. He was able to come back to himself and his own grounded sense of center. This was pretty new for Jonathon. He had lived outside of himself most of his life because of the events with his dad. Getting a felt, visceral sense of his own inner center or core was life-changing.

At the same time, we worked on using techniques of subtle body-building that helped Jonathon to further strengthen his ability to hold his own straightness and verticality no matter what was going on around him.

He was delighted with his full recovery and went off to pursue his dreams. In fact a couple of years later, he was instrumental in the field of cryptocurrencies as well as many other creative tech projects that went on to forge important pathways in the field of AI.

Part of the recovery for Jonathon, myself, and many others who got over CFS or burnout using subtle body-building, was learning and practicing uplifting.

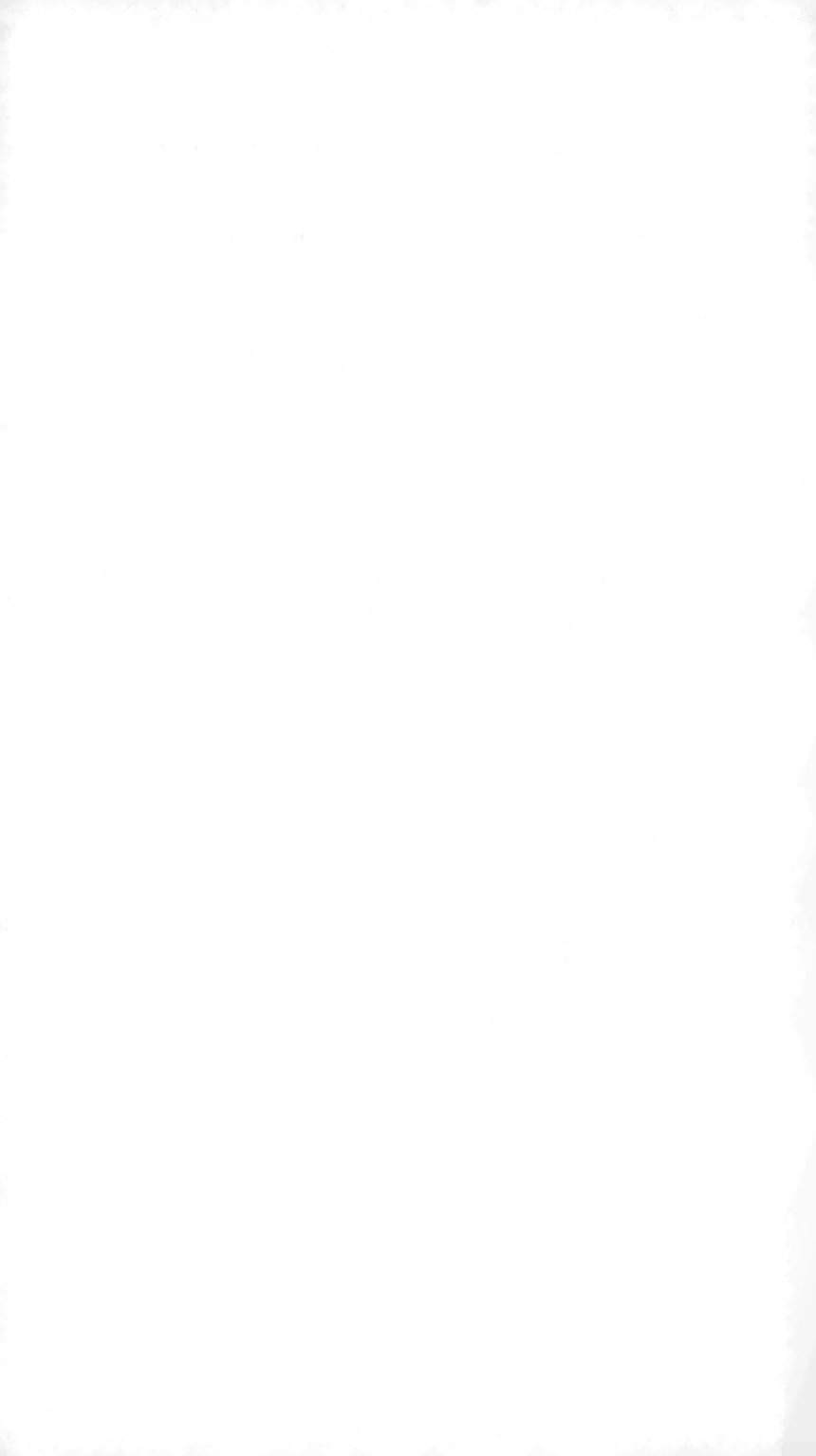

8

HARNESSING THE POWER OF NOBLE CHAOS (AND SLEEP)

Sleep is key at all phases of recovery, but telling you that good quality sleep and rest is paramount throughout recovery from CFS/ME, burnout or Long COVID, or even any kind of post-viral fatigue, is probably something you already know.

If you are like so many people that I have seen with these issues, then sleep and good quality rest are a struggle at the best of times. You might have insomnia, hypersomnia, or just wake up exhausted and unable to function through the day. Rest itself can be draining and boring, not delivering the level of rejuvenation that you need.

You are not alone. Many people with CFS, burnout, and Long COVID lose the ability to really let go in a way that allows regeneration and healing, including in the act of sleep.

So if sleep and good rest are so obviously key to the recovery of so many deeply exhausted and unwell people around the world, why haven't we worked out how to do it well?

Learning how to really let go and experience deep regeneration is one of the most important skills that I had to consciously regain through meditation and IST. It was absolutely key in my recovery from CFS and, later, from Long COVID.

Let's face it—learning how to sleep well is really a bit of a super power in this modern age. For me, cultivating the art of resting efficiently has been rewarding, pleasurable and key to my ability to get well and stay well. Honestly, it has also been paramount in my ability to be way more efficient in the whole of my life, including the waking parts.

Exploring sleep is really all about the mysterious power of yin states, the higher power of the feminine forces within us.

Therefore, having looked at the overexertion or overstimulation of our astral or more masculine side of the yinyang flow in the modern world, we now turn towards the inner world and the deepest mysteries hidden there. Of course sleep is the first step in this exploration because that is where we find the power of the night, the most yin aspects of our consciousness.

"Failed by the lack of public education, most of us do not realize how remarkable a panacea sleep truly is.... We will come to learn that sleep is the universal health care provider: whatever the physical, mental ailment, sleep has a prescription I can dispense."[55]

A good night of sleep is fast becoming a lost art. And a good night of sleep can be deeply healing and regenerative in so many ways, that without it our physical and mental wellbeing are in real jeopardy.

Through my own journey with CFS and Long COVID, I have learned how important good quality sleep is for any kind of recovery. The kind of sleep that makes you wake up feeling refreshed, vibrant, alive, and inspired is central to the process of getting better. I have learned to love a good sleep that brings dreams full of mystery and metaphor, filling up my heart and life force with buoyancy.

As fiction author Ben Okri says in the last line of his Nobel Prize-winning book *The Famished Road*, "A dream can be the highest point of a life."

What better way is there to "let go" than to have a good night of sleep? And our body of energy needs to let go in order to recover and heal. But what does it mean to let go?

---

55. Matthew P. Walker, *Why We Sleep: Unlocking the Power of Sleep and Dreams* (New York, NY: Scribner, an imprint of Simon & Schuster, Inc, 2018), 108.

SLEEP IN TERMS OF SUBTLE BODIES

"Sleep is not the absence of wakefulness. It is far more than that. Described earlier, our nighttime sleep is an exquisitely complex, metabolically active and deliberate series of unique stages."[56]

Exploring sleep further using the model of subtle bodies, it is possible to see that this (mostly) nocturnal activity is more than just a physical undertaking. There are a whole set of important mechanisms in the body of life force and our consciousness that are key for the "reboot" effect that comes from a good night of sleep.

When we lie down and nod off, our consciousness or astral body goes into more unconscious realms unrelated to the physical senses and the physical body. In this case, the life force, or etheric, our body of energy can let go and spread.[57]

Sleep can be seen as one of the ultimate examples of our life force, or the etheric body's yin or receptive power. Babies are a great example of this, sleeping anywhere, anytime, and waking up totally refreshed. Or have you ever seen a toddler have an over-tired tantrum and then almost fall over and just

---

56. Ibid.

57. Samuel Sagan, MD, *KT, Subtle Bodies, the Fourfold Model*, Point Horizon Institute, 2011, PDF for an audio recorded online correspondence course, 134.

sleep right there, waking up refreshed and light without a care in the world?

In contrast, perhaps you can relate to the observation that as many people get older, they lose the ability to drop in and stay in a deep refreshing state of sleep? This is largely because the etheric or the body of life force wears out as people age, and as a result it becomes increasingly challenging to let go into slumber in the way a small child does.

The good news is that you can learn to consciously let go into sleep, even as you age. This is part of the suite of techniques that help people recover from ongoing, unexplained fatigue.

Sleep is so mysterious to most of us. All we know is that when our head hits the pillow, we are supposed to drift off in less than a second without even realizing how it happens. Then with luck we seem to travel through the night, possibly visiting people, landscapes, images and deep spaces of unconsciousness, returning replenished and often with new ideas, new enthusiasm, and fresh health.

Sleeping like a child is often seen as a gift, almost as if it happens without any conscious involvement at all. This ability to totally let go into the fertile principle of the night is an active letting go of the waking state so that the body can go back to into horizontality and do what it needs to do for healing and rejuvenation.

When they sleep, children tend to dream, and their mind travels far away from the physical reality of their body. This allows the body of life force to spread and dive into the states of chaos like the ocean or a rich fertile earth.

As adults, many people lose that ability, but it can be relearned and cultivated with some meditative techniques and knowhow about what fosters the ability to let go in this way.

People are generally less able to let go as they get older because there is more of a tendency to grasp or hold onto inner tension. The astral body or principle of consciousness gets stronger, and the vehicle of life, the etheric, weakens.

Grasping can be triggered by things like underlying anxiety, tension, or just the wrong relationship with the life force through bad food and health.

But we do not have to be a slave to the norm. We can cultivate other functions in the etheric-astral balance inside of ourselves through meditation or other techniques.

Learning how to sleep properly is learning how to let go in a full and deep way back into the principle of life, which of course is not as easy as it sounds. Otherwise, the huge percentage of the adult population struggling with sleep would have figured it out.

However, from a standpoint of subtle bodies, it is simple. The state of consciousness that we are in during the day totally influences the quality of sleep that we have. So if we are in states of intense grasping and pushing all day long, with no opportunity to ebb and flow between yin and yang forces inside of ourselves, then it is very hard to become receptive to the power of sleep at night.

The intense grasping and stress of modern life does not promote good sleep at all.

MODERN LIFE DETRACTS FROM THE POWER OF NOBLE CHAOS

The materialist agenda of the modern world judges sleep a waste of time, undermining the potential immense healing power of sleep, and the return to source consciousness or this noble chaos. Our lives currently do very little to promote this important aspect of our energy and ourselves. Even more than that, our lives right now are set up to draw us out of this yin, healing, chaos of life force.

Take for example, the way that our digestive systems needs to break food down into chaos, illustrating how important these aspects of primordial life are in our bodies. Fermented foods like sauerkraut or other delicacies that feed our gut flora and living organic foods from soil have a tremendous healing power because they speak to a process that is meant to happen in our own guts. Our own stomachs and digestion include this fertile chaos as the principle of fermentation is so key to a healthy gut. Yet the increasing amount of processed food and chemicals in our diets gets in the way of the need for this process to happen in our bodies.

Sleep is no different. Our energy needs to return to this place of no grasping where there is a total release of tension and the noble chaos can take over, feeding us on many levels. But we are so overstimulated and stuck in intense states of tension and striving that we have forgotten how to let go.

Part of the power of chaos in the etheric is the ability to churn, or wash and mix our life force energies, lifting out the consciousness or astral aspect of our subtle bodies. Sleep is a time when we really let go of the tension, control, and gripping of the astral body to allow the etheric to churn. Meaning it is mixed and swirled, clarified and cleansed. Ideally in this process, there is an aspect of the astral body or our consciousness traveling to higher realms.

Sagan says:

How can you know if you have journeyed into high spheres during the night?

You feel fantastic in the morning. More than just a superior quality of rest, the experience is one of lightness of the soul.

Another sign is a certain high quality in the heart, a proper 'enthusiasm' (as in 'God inside'), which is an aftereffect of the great clarity experienced during the night. Carried by this enthusiasm, you are likely to be creative, at your peak of productivity.[58]

---

58. Ibid.

INSOMNIA AND OTHER SLEEP ISSUES, A BIGGER PROBLEM THAN CFS, LONG COVID, OR BURNOUT

People are exhausted, experiencing insomnia and other sleep issues like restless leg syndrome and even hypersomnia.

Walker describes how even with a strict clinical definition of insomnia, which is not the same as being sleep deprived, about one in nine people in America have this problem, *"which translates to more than 40 million Americans struggling to make it through their waking days due to wide-eyed nights."*

> *In truth, insomnia is likely to be a more widespread and serious problem than even these sizeable numbers suggest. Should you relax the stringent clinical criteria and just use epidemiological data as a guide, it is probably two out of every three people reading this book will regularly have difficulty falling or staying asleep at least one night a week, every week.*[59]

Many people struggle with letting go when they lie down to sleep. They struggle for a number of reasons. For a start, the mind is typically overstimulated during the day with

---

59. Matthew P. Walker, *Why We Sleep: Unlocking the Power of Sleep and Dreams* (New York, NY: Scribner, an imprint of Simon & Schuster, Inc, 2018), 242-243.

screens, phones, and other distractions, while the body has not been supported the way it needs to be with food and time in nature or good exercise. All of these factors leave people in a state of grasping.

Grasping or gripping or tension in the body is a physical result of the astral body grasping onto the etheric. When this is pushed too far, it just doesn't let go properly. Think of the hand holding onto a taut rope for a long time, and when it is time to let go, it stays tight and tense even though the job is done.

If you are up all night watching horror movies and depressing dramas, drinking beer and eating pizza, then when you finally lie down to sleep, your mind is still in those spaces of consciousness. Or if you spend all day wired on caffeine, anxious about your survival, gripped in an emotional or mental tension, then it can be harder to lift off and go on into a state of levity needed for the body of life to be able to spread and regenerate.

The key to being able to look after your body of energy and allow it to do what it needs to do when you are asleep is understanding that this is a body of rhythms. Just like a baby or a small child that benefits enormously from a good routine, the body of energy also loves a good routine that puts it in harmony with its own rhythmic nature.

When you put a baby to sleep, you do not play heavy metal music or make it watch violent video games. You create a quiet and restful space around the baby; you give it the things it needs to understand this is bedtime. The routine of bathtime, physical warmth and touch, soft lighting, and of course the things that help the child to feel safe all create an environment where they can let go.

There are a few things that really impact many people's sleep alongside the attention to rhythms, including energetic blockages that stop a person's body of life force from being able to let go at night. For example, a very small number of cases have something like an energetic parasite which really hampers any ability to let go and contributes significantly to CFS-type symptoms.

According to Samuel Sagan, MD, *"Entities exist, but they are not everywhere! Moreover one does not catch one without good reasons. So let us not develop an entity paranoia, or try to protect ourselves against something which, apart from exceptional cases, cannot touch us."*[60]

---

60. Samuel Sagan, *Entity Possession: Freeing the Energy Body of Negative Influences* (Rochester, Vt: Destiny Books, 1997), 188-189.

SLEEP AND CFS, LONG COVID

Sleep fights against infection and sickness by deploying all manner of weaponry within your immune arsenal, cladding you with protection. When you do fall ill, the immune system actively stimulates the sleep system, demanding more bed rest to help reinforce the war effort. Reduce sleep even for a single night, and that invisible suit of immune resilience is rudely stripped from your body.[61]

Many people with CFS or Long COVID, or even burnout have phases of both hypersomnia and insomnia. They also do not wake up feeling refreshed, but rather wake up feeling hungover, foggy, and tired even after hours of sleep.

Creyos (formerly Cambridge Brain Sciences), which leads the field when it comes to accurately quantifying brain function and brain health, says that for everyone, no matter how well or unwell they are, "lack of sleep can impair your brain as much as being intoxicated by alcohol."[62]

---

61. Matthew P. Walker, *Why We Sleep: Unlocking the Power of Sleep and Dreams* (New York, NY: Scribner, an imprint of Simon & Schuster, Inc, 2018), 181.

62. "Is Staying up Late Similar to Being Drunk?," Creyos, April 25, 2024, https://creyos.com/resources/articles/staying-up-late-same-as-being-drunk.

And oversleeping can also create symptoms of a hangover, even if you are physically fit. *"Oversleep causes a feeling similar to feeling hungover, and it's caused by the same biological function that gives you jet lag,"* says Nick Stockton.[63]

When I first had symptoms of CFS, I had been working night shifts for a phase, and then after finishing night shifts, I started experiencing hypersomnia, meaning I couldn't stop sleeping. My head would fall down towards my desk even at work, and on weekends I would be drawn to my bed for deep long naps all through the day. Anytime I put my head down, I would drift immediately into a deep soporific kind of sleep, full of dreams and rich imagery. I was constantly dragging myself out of these magnetic pulls towards sleep, pulling myself back to a waking (and dragging fatigued) state.

Looking back, when I was going into those deep rich states of dreaming, just putting my head on the desk (in an open-plan office), my body was trying to heal. I would not let it do that because I judged sleeping that way to be bad and lazy.

When I got COVID in 2022, even after I had spent years developing and cultivating my subtle bodies, I went down like a sack of potatoes. At first I slept, slept, slept a lot, because when I got CFS the first time I had made the mistake of not

---

63. Nick Stockton, "What's up with That: Why Does Sleeping in Just Make Me More Tired?," *Wired*, July 22, 2014, https://www.wired.com/2014/07/whats-up-with-that-why-does-sleeping-in-just-make-me-more-tired/.

sleeping enough, doubting my body, and pushing too hard. This time, I wanted to do the opposite.

When I first got sick with COVID, I slept 10, 15 or sometimes even 20 hours a day. Then after recovering from COVID, I had Long COVID for about five months. It was exhausting, and while I worked through most of it, I could not get a sense of being recovered, no matter how much I slept.

One of the big factors in recovery is knowing when to sleep and when to get up and move, to create a vertical momentum of engagement. It took me years to figure this out, and still I had to really place awareness on this to recover the second time.

The tricky part for me was not when I was really sick but when I was deeply fatigued but essentially better from the initial phase of the viral infection. This middle phase of the illness was where I was susceptible to overwork or over-rest, so I had to implement the understanding of active versus receptive modes throughout the day.

In the first stages of such an intense illness, rest can be absolutely key to recovery. True to my pattern of pushing too hard in my life, when I had COVID, I did rest for eight days, and then I got up and started working, in my impatience again missing that recovery from this illness was going to be different from other viruses. I was unwell with symptoms of Long COVID for about five months after that, and I had to re-implement everything that I had learned with CFS to fully recover again. Many people are ill with Long COVID for a lot longer than five months, and I must admit that I was disappointed that I had it at all. But my experience with CFS meant that I knew what was happening and addressed it accordingly, so that it did not turn into something longer term.

Instead of just lying there, waiting to get better, I would rest and sleep a lot and then get up and move. Even if I could only walk a little, perhaps around the block, I moved what I could. This way I began to build up strength.

As strength was gradually rebuilding, I started to implement a routine that worked for my body, involving work, meditation, very gentle exercise, and regular phases of resting.

SLEEP AS A HEALING TOOL
– ADDRESSING THE IMBALANCES

Matthew Walker, PhD in his book *Why We Sleep: Unlocking The Power of Sleep and Dreams*, says that *"humans are not sleeping the way nature intended. The number of sleep bouts, the duration of sleep, and when sleep occurs have all been comprehensively distorted by modernity."*[64]

> *...In general, these unrefreshed feelings that compel a person to fall back asleep midmorning, or require the boosting of alertness with caffeine, are usually due to individuals not giving themselves adequate sleep opportunity time—at least eight or nine hours in bed.....*

Walker then goes on to say,

You then carry that outstanding sleepiness balance throughout the following day. Also like a loan in arrears, this sleep debt will continue to accumulate. You cannot hide from it. The debt will roll over into the next payment cycle, and they next, and the next, producing a condition of prolonged, chronic sleep deprivation from one day to another. This outstanding sleep obligation results in a

---

64. Matthew P. Walker, *Why We Sleep: Unlocking the Power of Sleep and Dreams* (New York, NY: Scribner, an imprint of Simon & Schuster, Inc, 2018), 68.

feeling of chronic fatigue, manifesting in many forms of mental and physical ailments that are now rife throughout industrialized nations.[65]

Many people cannot really answer questions about how their body prefers to sleep because they have never given themselves the space to find out. They have never had the opportunity to just let their body dictate their rhythms for a while.

The incredible level of mental and substance stimulation that people are receiving means that they are separated out from the way that their body would like to move through its day, its month, its year. The substances and the overstimulation also result in not being able to let go. They cause grasping, tension, agitation, wakefulness, or just plain old bad quality of sleep.

Sleep rhythms are badly impacted by the numerous stimulants and mind-altering substances that people have access to now, so that even when people lie down and do sleep, there is not a proper letting go. The mind is under the influence of buzzing phones, flashing computers, blaring TV screens, caffeine, alcohol, and sleeping pills, among other things, so that many people miss the opportunity to rest and let go properly.

In terms of subtle bodies, when the body lies down to sleep, the mind is meant to let go. Sometimes you might feel a

---

65. Matthew P. Walker, *Why We Sleep*, 36.

sense of this, like the feeling of lifting off, or flying or dropping back into the body when you wake up in a jolt. As you sleep the mind is only very distantly connected to the senses, as if it goes off on its own journey. During that time, the body of life force also is supposed to spread and go through a whole process of restoration that is deeply nourishing to us on every level. No more holding on or gripping or tension, just total release. In that release there is a lot done to regenerate and rejuvenate. Movements in the body of energy to cleanse, purify, and heal.

When we go to sleep, the life force energy is supposed to return to a kind of noble chaos. Chaos is defined by Merriam-Webster dictionary as "a state of utter confusion" or "a confused mass or mixture," "a state of things in which chance is supreme, especially the confused unorganized state of primordial matter before the creation of distinct forms."[66]

And noble in this case is referring to "possessing very high or excellent properties" as in "noble wine."[67] What's more, the fact this form of chaos is full of knowing, or the ability to know, is illustrated in the etymology of the word *noble* or its original meaning dating back to 1200, when it meant both "of superior birth" and literally "knowable" from the root *gno* "to know."

---

66. "Chaos Definition & Meaning," *Merriam-Webster*, accessed June 11, 2024, https://www.merriam-webster.com/dictionary/chaos.

67. "Noble Definition & Meaning," *Merriam-Webster*, accessed June 11, 2024, https://www.merriam-webster.com/dictionary/noble.

Noble chaos is a higher principle of chaos that churns our energy in a way that is healing and even brings inspiration. The ocean is a living example of noble chaos, its healing powers nourishing us whenever we visit. Or the tilling of the Earth before we sow the seeds, emphasizing the importance of chaos in the fertility cycle.

APHRODITE AND NOBLE CHAOS

The power of chaos and the feminine forces of nature are pointed to throughout mythology, where we have explored human beings' mixed relationship with those forces, both desiring the sensuality and requiring the fencing in of these primordial aspects of our consciousness for fear of losing ourselves.

Venus or Aphrodite is one of those ancient symbols of beauty, life, the feminine, sexuality, and the primordial forces of chaos that has spoken to much of humankind across centuries, according to Bettany Hughes in her book, *Venus and Aphrodite, A History of a Goddess*:

> *"Venus–or Aphrodite as she was originally called by the Greeks–was a primordial creature, said to have been born out of an endless black night before the beginning of the world."*

Hughes goes on to share the well-known myth that Aphrodite was said to be born out of the ocean after Kronos hacked off his father's erect penis and threw the "dismembered phallus and testicles into the sea."

"Rising up from her mother sea. Look,
The Cyprian, she whom Apelles laboured hard to paint?
How she takes hold of her tresses
Damp from the sea! How she wrings out the foam
From these wet locks of hers! Now Athene and Hera
Will say
In beauty we can never compete!"[68]

Hughes points out that human relationship with the forces of the feminine principles such as sexuality, life, beauty, and nature can be mapped through the way that different epochs depicted and referred to Venus and Aphrodite. While she has been worshipped and adored, she has also been looked down upon and cast aside as less than in many eras, including the current one.

The way that we flirt with our fear of primordial chaos and the power of the night was depicted in mythology by a less famous ancient Greek goddess Nyx, associated with night, and considered to be the daughter of Chaos.

---

68. Bettany Hughes, *Venus and Aphrodite: A Biography of Desire* (New York: Basic Books, 2020), 1.

Nyx, in Greek mythology, female personification of night but also a great cosmogonical figure, feared even by Zeus, the king of the gods, as related in Homer's Iliad, Book XIV. According to Hesiod's Theogony, she was the daughter of Chaos and the mother of numerous primordial powers, including Sleep, Death, the Fates, Nemesis, and Old Age.[69]

Also the domain of the night, there are issues such as energetic parasites or entities that deeply impact the articulation of life versus consciousness in our subtle bodies, and therefore make it difficult to let go into sleep. These are in the category of problems that really do need to be revealed through an exploration using a technique such as IST, and occasionally require healing or clearing therapy.

---

69. "Nyx," Encyclopædia Britannica, May 20, 2024, https://www.britannica.com/topic/Nyx.

CASE STUDY - LISA & AN ENERGETIC PARASITE, BLOCKING THE HEALING POWER OF SLEEP

When Lisa walked in the door, she filled the room with her golden sunny energy, her blonde curly hair, her big warm smile, her Botticelli figure. She was a young actor from South Africa, looking for a way to recover from CFS. I met Lisa when I was working as an IST practitioner in London, UK. She had gotten sick 18 months before, when she was 25 years old in her home town in Johannesburg, South Africa.

She was a very warm, outgoing, bubbly person, but when she was 25 years old, she had been held up at gunpoint at night in a parking lot by a group of young African males. They took her car and valuables when she was on her way home from a shift working in a nearby restaurant. After that, she collapsed and was in bed for several weeks. And the 18 months since were a horror show of symptoms that she had never had before, such as constant unexplained levels of fatigue, headaches, stomach issues, to the point that it was jeopardizing her career as an actor.

Since the event, she had been absolutely exhausted, and her sleep was awful, every single night. She woke up most of the time feeling hungover and beaten up.

She had been to see doctors, specialists and alternative healers in her home town Johannesburg and in London, UK, but so far nothing had really helped her to recover.

When we did the IST sessions, Lisa saw for herself that the shock of the incident where she was held up and robbed had created an ongoing tension in her body and energy that meant she could not let go properly. She saw that she was in a constant, unconscious state of anxiety and grasping. In addition, the severity of the shock had created a breach considerable enough that a foreign energy had entered her system. It had been acting like a parasite since, draining her and stopping her from really being able to let go and heal.

Very occasionally, I have seen people who have picked up an energetic parasite bad enough to drain the person's vitality, stop them from sleeping in a way that is refreshing, and even prove toxic enough to create serious health issues. Lisa was one of those people.

Just as there are physical parasites that can seriously affect people's health and wellbeing, there are also nonphysical or energetic parasites that potentially contribute to CFS, among other things.

When Lisa caught the parasite, she was in a state of shock, and completely ungrounded. In her terror from the event, she had unknowingly allowed something to enter her subtle bodies that would not otherwise have been able to get in. Her energy was unusually breached because of the shocking level of the holdup.

Many people have something of a freeze response when unexpectedly thrown into a deep trauma, which means that their consciousness is slightly withdrawn or retracts from the body. They are no longer grounded in their body in that moment, dissociated, allowing a kind of energetic breach.

This lack of grounded awareness leaves a kind of gap or rupture momentarily between the consciousness and the vitality in the body, and that is when people are potentially more susceptible to some kind of foreign energy entering their system.

The Clairvision School uses the term 'entity' for these parasitic energies. The founder Sagan says in the introduction of his book *Entity Possession: Freeing the Energy Body of Negative Influences*:

> *The term entity refers to nonphysical beings, presences which become attached to human beings and act as parasites, thereby creating various emotional, mental and physical problems ranging from eating disorders and uncontrollable emotions to the most severe disease.*[70]

Sagan's book is a great reference for understanding a systematic approach to exploring and removing entities as it is done with IST.

The point here is that there are a few cases where people like Lisa have a particularly nasty and rare kind of energetic parasite or entity, which actually creates something that looks

---

70. Samuel Sagan, *Entity Possession: Freeing the Energy Body of Negative Influences* (Rochester, Vt: Destiny Books, 1997), 1.

like CFS and makes the letting-go aspect of sleep impossibly difficult.

Lisa was such a bubbly and joyful person that the starting point of her illness was pretty distinct. She was not sick before she was held up in the parking lot that night. And yet her symptoms would not respond to Western medicine or alternative therapies until she came to see me.

After we used IST to separate out and clear the parasitic energy that was plaguing her, Lisa let me know that she was completely better. Part of the process of separation involved releasing the trauma and emotional charge from the incident of the attack, allowing a lot of healing beyond having the fragment removed. It had a profoundly positive effect on her life, she said.

She kindly wrote me a thank-you letter about a year later letting me know that she had not had any CFS symptoms since the clearing.

Catching one of these entities or parasites is not a common occurrence. It can happen in a situation where someone is unconscious, where they are in shock, or where something has happened to create an unusual level of breach. And among the rare cases that someone catches such a perverse energy, it is even rarer that it would cause something as severe as CFS.

Sagan points out that the topic of entities or parasites of energy is both old and new.

Old, because in all traditions and folklores of the earth, one finds references to spirits and nonphysical beings which can interfere with human beings. Thus Ayurveda, the traditional medicine of India, is divided into eight sections, one of which is entirely devoted to the study of bhūtas, or entities, their influence on health and sanity, and the ways one can get rid of them.[71]

Interestingly, Sagan says that this means Ayurveda places the 'science of entities' on the same level as surgery or gynecology.

And in Chinese medicine, this topic historically was also a common part of the healing practices, Sagan points out: *"If we look at traditional Chinese medicine, we find that in acupuncture, among the 361 points of the 14 main meridians, 17 have the word Kuei (disincarnate spirit) as part of their secondary name."*[72]

Part of the technique of IST is that practitioners never tell the client what they see in a way that would block their own experience. Thus when I worked with Lisa for example, I did not mention that there might be a parasite of energy. Rather, I guided her into the inner space through the meditation technique and helped her to see what was happening in her own energy.

---

71. Ibid.

72. Ibid.

Once they have the techniques of IST and a practitioner, clients like Lisa do not have to know what a parasite is to see it inside of themselves. Usually when they see this kind of blockage in their body, they know pretty quickly that it doesn't feel right and that it is not them. Once they have the context, they are pretty happy to explore it and get it removed.

One of the things that entities can really interrupt is the subtle body processes of sleep. When a person has a parasitic energy, it acts a bit like a stone in their subtle bodies, weighing everything down so that the proper takeoff of consciousness from the life force cannot happen. This on its own can be deeply depleting. But if the parasite is also sucking the life force and even polluting it with its own toxic gunk, illness can result. And sometimes that looks like CFS, although it is rarely the sole cause of the illness.

9

WHAT CAN YOU DO TO RECOVER THE REFRESHING POWER OF SLEEP?

The constant ebb and flow of yin and yang throughout our inner and outer worlds shows us that these two states are deeply interconnected. In fact they are really two sides of the same coin—our own state of being and the universe around us.

That deep interconnectedness of the yin and yang motions through day and night illustrates that the states of consciousness that you are in during the day completely influence the states that you enter in the night.

INTERNALIZATION VERSUS EXTERNALIZATION

Accordingly, in the hour or so before your nighttime slumber, it is important to have some kind of internalization, so that consciousness has a good trajectory for letting go.

There are different types of fatigue in terms of subtle bodies, and each can have a different result regarding our ability to rest. There is the simple example of the etheric or the body of life force just being depleted from a day of work. Life force was not designed to sustain activity forever. It needs to stop and recuperate as we have already established.

But then you can also have a kind of tiredness that is more from the astral body, like an emotional or stress fatigue. Sagan points out in the online audio recorded correspondence course, *Knowledge Track: Flow of Life,* that stress is exhausting because in this state the astral body squeezes the etheric and its essential energies. This is a kind of externalization of consciousness that results in a particular kind of tiredness.

> *"There is only so much of this the etheric body can take,"* Sagan says of stress. *"Same with high anxiety and intense emotions. If out of control, the constant astral grasping will dry out the etheric body."*[73]

---

73. Samuel Sagan, MD, *KT Flow of Life*, Point Horizon Institute, 2011, from the written PDF for audio recordings on an online correspondence course, 76.

Sagan talks about the type of exhaustion that people with CFS experience as a third and different type of tiredness.

With CFS the etheric body finds itself under the constant, exhausting pressure of astral intensity. This has a lot to do with the modern lifestyle: stress and all sorts of factors that raise intensity in the astral body. The astral constantly grasps and wears out the etheric, resulting in exhaustion.[74]

The thing is that this third type of exhaustion is really hard to recover from. It is not usually something that a night of sleep will fix because once someone is in that state of chronic depletion, they really struggle to let go in the way that is needed for a truly regenerative rest. This type of letting go only happens when we can take that over externalized grasping of the astral body and turn it back, like turning our consciousness inside out. This comes from a deep internalization of consciousness.

Internalization can mean time off screens, or dimming the lights, or quiet time reading, and being with loved ones in the hour before bed. Sometimes for me, it can also mean gentle very quiet yoga exercises a short meditation, or a gentle walk in a park through nature as part of unwinding from the day, essentially bringing the externalization of the yang orientation of consciousness back inside.

---

74. Samuel Sagan, MD, *KT Flow of Life*, 77.

YINYANG MOVEMENTS THROUGHOUT THE DAY

One of the things that I learned was to have some kind of rhythm or yinyang flow throughout the day. What I mean is allowing my body to sleep when it really needed it, even if that was longer than I judged it should be, and getting up to implement gentle exercise and movement to create the yang motion too. This flow and rhythm is the opposite of the stagnation of sitting in a car, behind a desk, in front of the television, and so on.

Life force is a body of rhythms; it likes to flow, and it loves routines. Babies illustrate this well. They respond so well to routines and rhythms that when you throw them out for a day, moving their nap times or relocating them, it can take frazzled parents days to get the child back on track with sleep patterns.

There are natural times during the day when each person has stronger or weaker energy. For example, mornings versus afternoons can be pretty different for most people. A mid-afternoon nap of about 20 minutes has been shown to be beneficial for many people.[75]

I found too that it was important for me to implement a (fluid) routine in my sleep patterns after meeting Ray, an

---

75. Matthew Walker, "Matthew Walker's Defense of Napping: 5 Benefits of Napping - 2024," MasterClass, June 7, 2021, https://www.masterclass.com/articles/matthew-walkers-defense-of-napping.

acupuncturist in Sydney, Australia who was well-known for helping people with CFS to recover. What I mean is that I was never too rigid about it, but I tried to be in bed before 10 p.m. and awake by 7 a.m. This rhythm worked for me as I am someone who is an early riser, usually up around 6:30 a.m.

Ray helped many people who had spent a year or more in bed to recover, he told me. He shared with me extensively about the importance of getting back into healthy sleep rhythms in order to recover from CFS. He said that many of his clients got stuck with CFS because they were staying up very late at night and getting up late in the day, and this totally screwed their innate ability to follow the rhythms of their body.

Ray would ask his clients to create a routine around their sleep patterns, encouraging them to wake up and go to sleep at similar times, having a rhythm. This approach to bringing the body back into harmony with its own rhythms really helped a number of his clients recover from CFS, he said.

PHASES OF RECOVERY AND SLEEP PATTERNS

From what I have observed in my own energy and the experience of clients, the sleep routine needed in recovery from CFS and Long COVID can vary at different phases of the illness.

Initially, when sick with the infection, there is a huge need to sleep way more than the ordinary mind might deem reasonable.

After a few weeks, when the next phase towards recovery begins, there is a real need to establish a steady pattern of sleeping and waking. Meaning that there is a gentle routine established of waking hours and sleeping hours, with rest times of 30 to 60 minutes once or twice a day as needed.

The etheric body is a body of rhythms, and it responds well to routines, just as babies respond well to routines. This is because their consciousness is almost completely resting on the energy of life force as they have very few astral or thoughts and emotions impacting them.

The more your etheric recovers its ability to let go and rejuvenate, the more you will benefit from these gentle rhythms between waking and sleeping hours, with regular rest periods structured into your day.

Let's talk a little more about the art of resting well during the day.

PROMOTING NOBLE CHAOS
THROUGH NIGHT PRACTICE

Conquering the art of noble chaos in my own body of energy was about coming into alignment with its rhythms, and riding them rather than fighting against them.

In those first nine months after meeting Ruth-Helen, my life changed dramatically. I went from being on social welfare, working as a volunteer senior support person, to going back into a part-time job in journalism, then a job as an editor of a finance magazine, and finally starting my own business as a freelance journalist.

I went from crashing all the time, spending about two-thirds of my days in bed unable to work, to getting back to part-time work and spending my days off in bed. Building my strength until within six months I was back at full-time work, with very little residue of the CFS. Within eighteen months, all residues of the illness were gone.

As part of this very fast suite of positive changes, I moved out of a pretty old and musty place that was not helping my energy at all into a new house that backed onto a national park in Lane Cove, Sydney NSW. The house was surrounded by a forest of deep, lush green trees and ferns. I lived with a handful of eccentric new friends there, while starting out my own business as a freelance writer.

I was in recovery and stepping out of my comfort zone, including a totally new way to manage the CFS illness and symptoms. Sometimes, though, I would still get exhausted or find it hard to make it through the day, or even crash for a day or two. Ruth-Helen would often help me with a session or a phone call to walk me through what had pulled me down, and help me to get back up on my feet again.

One of the most practical tools that I used at that time to recover was the "night practice." This is a lying-down meditative practice that deeply restores and nourishes the body of vitality and also provides creative inspiration and even spiritual regeneration.

Once I was working at home, I would work hard for several hours researching and preparing several articles at a time. It was the days of dial-up internet so there was some time spent downloading web pages for research. During this time, I would do some mini dynamic meditation exercises to keep myself alert and awaken.

When I had done all I could to gather my material, and I was exhausted, I would do what I never did before. I would lie down, but not just lay down, but do a short horizontal meditative practice.

It was so beautiful. A total letting go into the horizontality, surfing the edge between being asleep and awake. Even if that practice was just 15 minutes long because I was on a very tight deadline, I would emerge completely refreshed and often find the work a lot faster and smoother to complete than it would have been if I had remained sitting at my desk, pushing myself through.

This is such a great example of working with our own inner rhythms. In those first phases of recovery from CFS, I would often do a few of those lying-down practices in a day so that by the end of the day, I was not in pain, not dragging myself from one activity to another, not tight and gripped with physical fatigue. I would go to bed and be able to fully surrender into the bliss of a really good night of sleep.

Attuning ourselves to the rhythms or the changes in life is something that happens through the practices of meditation-based techniques over time. My experience is that my consciousness became more and more functional on increasingly subtle levels of existence. At the same time, I learned to utilize surrender, as well as the fight and the push. I learned to be receptive, letting things come to me and also to get up and work to make things happen.

It is easy to see how the cycle of birth and death has a rhythm to it, but that same cycle happens for us every single day, waking up, living our day, and then going to sleep like a mini death. This is so important in our consciousness that the ancient and most revered Indian text of the Bhagavad-Gita points to it:

In that which is night to all beings,
the enlightened one is awake.
That in which all beings are awake,
is night to the enlightened one.
Bhagavad-Gita 2.69

There are three chapters about night practice in the book *Awakening The Third Eye* by Samuel Sagan, MD. There, he writes in detail about the parallel between the moment of dying and the moment of falling asleep. The states of consciousness that you visit during sleep influence the quality of your rest.

> *A whole range of planes of consciousness are open to you. Some are light and refreshing; others are more likely to induce nightmares. As far as fatigue recovery and spiritual development are concerned, sleep quality depends on the quality of the planes that your astral body visits during the night. If you wander into the wrong places, you may well wake up more tired than when you fell asleep or even sick... At the gate of sleep, as at the gate of death, a resonance takes place. At the very moment of falling asleep, the quality of your consciousness plays an essential role in determining where you will journey during the night.*[76]

Why is it so powerful? Night practice is so powerful because it is using the interface between being awake and asleep. Interfaces are places where our consciousness cannot hang on.

Take another powerful interface, dawn or dusk. Many people have had spiritual awakenings at either dawn or dusk,

---

76. Samuel Sagan MD, *Awakening the Third Eye* (Roseville, N.S.W, Australia: Clairvision, 1997), 163.

including the Buddha who is said to have become enlightened at dawn after a night of fighting off the demons or maras under the Bodhi Tree.

> *Siddhartha then continued with his meditation until dawn, when he attained the varja-like concentration. With this concentration, which is the very last mind of a limited being, he removed the final veils of ignorance from his mind and in the next moment became a Buddha, a fully enlightened being.*[77]

My experience of doing these night practices regularly throughout the day was that my subtle bodies began to change. Where I would usually push into fatigue, and create a major pathway of grasping, a precursor to crashing, I began to learn to surrender to the light of spiritual realms. My subtle bodies became more flexible, more supple, more able to hold the fire of vertically pressing into projects and work.

I also became a lot better at recovery. I learned that when I crashed, I could use this ability to surf the interface between sleeping and waking as a conscious tool to rejuvenate myself much more quickly than I had in the past.

Another benefit that totally surprised me was that I became a lot quicker at my job. This might sound strange, but I learned to use the interface between waking and sleeping to

---

77. "Buddha's Enlightenment," Kadampa Buddhism, March 13, 2023, https://kadampa.org/reference/buddhas-enlightenment).

work on projects in a way that was full of surrender. When I was writing an article, and I got stuck, I would lie down for a 15- or 20-minute meditative rest, and let go of whatever it was that I was pushing up against. More often than not, while I was lying down, resting, a creative solution or a packed knowing of the very thing that I was working on would come to me. When I got up to address it, it just flowed out of me without any "friction-ful" thinking and worrying. What a breeze!

GOOD ENERGY IN THE ROOM & HOUSE WHERE YOU SLEEP (INCLUDING EARTH LINES)

The environment in which we sleep deeply informs the quality of rest that we can have. For instance, I make sure that I do not have any screens in my bedroom when I go to bed. My computer, phone, and tablet are either in another room or turned off at night, reducing the interference of electromagnetic frequencies.

I usually make the room that I sleep in just for sleeping and meditating, so that my body of energy knows that this is a place where it can go internal and really let go. There is an aura of peace in my environment.

"Bad things happen in bad places," said Sagan.

But how do you know if it is a bad place?

When you create a room for a baby to sleep in, you make it conducive to restful sleep, peace and quiet. When you walk into a room where a baby sleeps, you hope to feel that sense of lightness, a good feeling, as if it were a place where you would like to rest yourself.

It is so helpful for the quality of our sleep, just like a baby, to have a peaceful space and good energy.

How do you know if a room has a good energy for sleeping? Sit quietly in that room, and ask yourself—how do you feel? Do you want to let go? Do you feel that it is clean and supportive? You will very quickly know whether it's a good place for sleep or not.

Learning to meditate with the third eye opens the perception of subtle energies of spaces. When you have meditated for a few weeks or months, and your inner vision is opening, there is a pathway to see for yourself what kind of space your bedroom and your house has.

But even before that, most people know when a room feels heavy and dark as opposed to light and inviting. It is quite instinctual to walk into a place and sense whether you would feel comfortable sleeping there.

EARTH LINES AND THE ENERGY OF YOUR BEDROOM

I had one client who had CFS for a number of years. He was drained and exhausted all the time. He had his house assessed by someone who could sense the energy of the space and found out that there were a lot of unusual energy lines in that house.

It was located in a place where the local earth energies were unusually toxic, heavy, and seemed to be attracting sickness. He tried to use crystals and all sorts of things to make it better. But in the end, he and his wife sold the house and found something in a much better location. His sleep quality improved, his energy improved, and he got better from CFS.

Checking out the energy of a place that you live or work can be done through sensing earth lines. These are lines that run like a grid around the earth and seem to concentrate negative energies. They are part of the earth, like meridians are part of the human body of life, and they have their place in the overall energetic environment of the earth. But it can be harmful to people's health to sleep, meditate, or spend long hours sitting on them.

"The lines, and especially the more noxious ones, seem to concentrate negative energies. This effect is at maximum intensity where the lines intersect. In other words, in a room the lines act like

energetic trash cans and gather 'etheric dirt,'" says Samuel Sagan, MD, in the book, *Awakening the Third Eye.*

Sagan continues:

Nobody really knows the exact nature of these lines. The term 'earth rays' is unfortunate and misleading: even though the whole phenomenon appears as some form of telluric radiation, no actual 'rays' have ever been identified.... As far as third eye vision is concerned, these earth lines do not appear so much as lines but more like walls.[78]

Most houses and homes can be improved through things like clutter clearing, a new paint job, reducing the EMFs, finding the best place to put your bed, and even having professionals come in to clear the space. However, there are a few places that are just not really fit for human habitation, and there is not a lot that we can do about it.

I once went to a house in Melbourne, Victoria in what used to be the red-light district there. I had been asked to go to clear some noxious energies. This is a simple procedure, except when there is an underlying issue in the area of the house that cannot really be changed.

This house was in an area where there were many perverse energies floating around, but they were not the real

---

78. Samuel Sagan MD, *Awakening the Third Eye* (Roseville, N.S.W, Australia: Clairvision, 1997), 163.

cause of the problem. The real cause of the problem was what had attracted all of that stuff in the first place, the underlying wrongness in that little area of the town.

It was just a few city blocks where there was something extremely toxic in the underlying earth energies. I would not recommend that anyone live somewhere like that. It is the kind of place that you are better off selling and moving on because the impact on the health of the inhabitants can be severe.

Living in a place like that could certainly give a person something like CFS or other severe health and psychological issues. It is not a space that is conducive to good sleep.

This is rare, though. Most places are good enough to be cleared or fixed up so that they become conducive to good sleep and healing, or rest.

ELECTROMAGNETIC FIELDS (EMFs)

EMFs are part of our lives, particularly living in an urban environment. They are a physical frequency resulting from technology including wireless, cell phones, computers, televisions, and other electronic devices. The studies are mixed as to whether or not EMFs impact the quality of sleep, and that is because the things that are impacted are on the level of life force. They are not physical. There is no specific biological marker that indicates the presence of EMFs. But by affecting the life force, EMFs are negatively impacting the quality of sleep, preventing the full letting go that is so healing.

The best thing to do is to see for yourself. Check to see if your sleep quality is better when you take all technology out of your room and ensure that you are not sleeping near to the power box if it is located outside of your house.

Give yourself three weeks of sleeping without anything in your room or nearby that can elevate EMFs. Take a journal each day and note down the hours of sleep, how you felt when you woke up, and whether you felt it made a difference to be sleeping with fewer EMFs in your environment.

A study conducted in Iran of workers at substations exposed to ELFMF (Extremely Low Frequency-Magnetic Field) showed,

> *...a positive correlation coefficient between occupational exposures to ELF electromagnetic fields and sleep quality score, so it cannot reject the impact of the fields on sleep quality. Since other finding indicated the weak electromagnetic fields can have the biological effects and reducing work hours can prevent their biological effects.*
>
> *Finally, exposure to electromagnetic fields or EMF has raised concern on the possible health effects of them; therefore they have become an interest issue for a great number of people (especially people who live near power lines) and are an active area of biophysical research; but*

for providing more accurate results, much more research is needed.[79]

GOOD DIET, EAT LIGHT IN THE EVENING & NOT TOO LATE

Look, I have been as neurotic as the next person about food, following all sorts of crazy diets trying to improve my health symptoms. Fasting, allergy diets, keto, paleo, vegan, macrobiotic, and more. It can go on and on. In the end, I really like the premise of eating food that is full of life force in a way that makes my body feel good and improves my health.

Use your own self-knowledge to figure out the best diet for you. Keep it as simple as possible and eat for life.

As I am not a nutritionist nor an expert in diet, I really cannot begin to advise anyone on what to eat or when they should eat it, but just say that finding the right balance for you does make a really big difference. Separate out knowing what your body needs from all of the unnecessary neurosis that can come from the many approaches to diet and nutrition freely available online.

---

79. Tayebeh Barsam et al., "Effect of Extremely Low Frequency Electromagnetic Field Exposure on Sleep Quality in High Voltage Substations," Iranian journal of environmental health science & engineering, November 30, 2012, https://www.ncbi.nlm.nih.gov/pmc/articles/PMC3561068/.

A diet that is healthy for you is important because conditions for good sleep quality are the same conditions for good health. Eat food that is alive, mostly plant-based, and locally grown when possible, and you will feed your body with life force, making it easier for sleep to nurture and nourish your body.

Eating late, eating a lot of sugar and caffeine, drinking alcohol, or taking mind-altering substances of any kind (whether recreational or prescribed) will impact the body's ability to regenerate and refresh itself in sleep.

> *Caffeine—which is not only prevalent in coffee, certain teas, and many energy drinks, but also foods such as dark chocolate and ice cream, as well as drugs such as weight-loss pills and pain relievers—is one of the most common culprits that keep people from falling asleep easily and sleeping soundly thereafter, typically masquerading as insomnia, an actual medical condition. Also be aware that de-caffeinated does not mean non-caffeinated. One cup of decaf usually contains 15 to 30 percent of the dose of a regular cup of coffee, which is far from caffeine-free, Walker says.*[80]

---

80. Matthew P. Walker, *Why We Sleep: Unlocking the Power of Sleep and Dreams* (New York, NY: Scribner, an imprint of Simon & Schuster, Inc, 2018), 29.

Walker talks about a "caffeine crash" where energy levels plummet, and it is difficult to function and concentrate, with strong pulls of sleepiness. On the physical side, this is because the caffeine blocks the sleepiness chemical—adenosine—but that same chemical builds up so that when the caffeine wears off, there is a crash.

Noble chaos has an elegance to it, a rhythm like that of the ocean, the moon cycle, the beneficial result of which is found in things like fermented foods which heal our gut. But when we have substances like caffeine, alcohol, marijuana, speed, or even LSD, that chaos becomes far from noble— more like chaotic mess than the beautiful fertile chaos. It is fallen and resonant with illness.

Walker illustrates this point well with the example of esoteric research conducted in the 1980s by NASA, giving spiders different drugs and then observing the webs they constructed. *"Researchers noted how strikingly incapable the spiders were in constructing anything resembling a normal logical web that would be of any functional use when given caffeine, even relative to the other potent drugs tested."*[81]

---

81. Matthew P. Walker, *Why We Sleep*, 30.

EXERCISE & STRETCHING
SO THE BODY CAN LET GO

There is mental exhaustion and physical exhaustion, and they feel different. The thing about mental exhaustion is that you feel fried and tired, but in that state the body has a hard time letting go.

After a day of mental stimulation, some time outside doing light exercise, or even more intense exercise if you are healthy, will help the body to let go.

Take a normally healthy group of people to the country and get them to do some hard labor, like chopping wood, digging ditches, building a basic shed or outdoor structure, or even gardening. Give them enough physical labor that their bodies are tired at the end of the day, and their minds are no longer holding onto anything. Let them breathe the fresh country air all day, smell the earth, listen to the sounds of birds and the breeze and the insects around them. And then ask them all about the quality of sleep that they have. You might find that most of them sleep more soundly than they do at home in their own urban environments when they spend most of their day online in one form or another.

Exercise can be very difficult for people with CFS or Long COVID because many have post-exertional malaise (PEM), meaning that their symptoms can dramatically worsen with exercise. I remember when I was so unwell and going for a short swim (two or three laps of the pool) would take me down for a week, although in my teens I easily swam for hours at a time training for competition.

There are treatments that include very small incremental steps to introducing exercise for someone with CFS/ME. I did use that approach to some degree in my own recovery, but I found that the timing and the awareness of where my body was at on any given day were really key to making it work.

I applied the "40 percent capacity rule" to my own return to exercise and knew that sometimes I would end up in bed. I got that rule from a chiropractor who helped me with a different physical injury. So for example, when I had a shoulder injury, totally unrelated to CFS, the chiropractor said to me, "Exercise at 40 percent of your capacity, and if you get injured or hurt the shoulder again, then stop until it is totally better and start at a further reduced capacity." I applied the same theory when recovering from CFS and later with Long COVID too, as part of a much bigger strategy, and I found that it really did work.

Studies do show a mixed response to incremental steps in returning to physical exercise, so people with these illnesses really need to monitor their own progress and see what works for them in the department of exercise. However, whatever happens, there is a need to move the body each day to reduce mental and emotional fatigue if at all possible.

In the case of mental fatigue, even a short phase of gentle stretching before going to bed can markedly improve sleep quality.

Moving to expel the exhaustion from the body is not really about fitness; it is more about moving the get the astral tension out of the body, freeing the muscles and the mind to be able to sleep properly.

If the fatigue is so bad that exercise really does bring you down further, then just see if you can get into nature every day. Get outside as an experiment, taking a break in nature, and see how your sleep quality changes or not.

Find ways to be in nature moving your body every day and see if this helps the quality of your sleep. Depending on your physical state, can you have regular smaller doses of the same thing in your daily life, gardening, walking in nature, or spending time outside doing small manual tasks?

To conclude, the yin power of sleep is essential for everyone, and the ability to rest well even for short naps during the day is deeply rejuvenating. Learning how to do this well is key for recovery from CFS/ME, burnout, and Long COVID.

10

WILLPOWER AND RECOVERING THE HEALTHY CREATIVE FLOW OF LIFE

The final phases of recovery for anyone with CFS/ME, burnout, Long COVID, or other types of illness resulting from crashing or collapsing in the subtle bodies are key. This is when you can build your life and your strength in a way that brings joy, wellness, and clarity.

For this next phase of recovery, and in the spirit of the yinyang symbol, we will turn back to the yang side of things and look at willpower. Moving into recovery and making it a reality in your life, it is key to be able to engage the fire of action in a positive way, in a way that does not burn you out.

The best possible scenario in the recovery from CFS and burnout is where someone is grounded in themselves such that they can start to execute willpower in a truly invigorating and inspiring way. This kind of engagement brings energy, even if you get tired at the end of each day. There is an uplift that comes through being on the right track for you and inspired in a flow.

To understand something about willpower, think of a newly-in-love couple, just starting out their relationship, who live across town from each other. They will stay up all night if needed, driving to or from each other's place, and work the next day without too much of a problem. The newly-in-love couple do things that ordinarily seem very difficult or nearly impossible because they have more energy ignited by the level of wanting or desire to be together. They are driven by the desire or the wanting that comes from their "in-love" state.

Wanting or desire is a driver for yang-style engagement. It makes people achieve an awful lot.

Yet so many clients who come to see me about CFS or burnout have lost touch with what they really want and as a result are very ungrounded in themselves, meaning they are not anchored in their own body and energy at all, but are living a life in their heads and outside of themselves.

Being ungrounded means having little or no direct experience of yourself and your feelings inside of your body, even if you do a lot of exercise, or get a lot done in your life.

Being ungrounded can result in draining the life force or vital energy. This is because the very engine of the body of energy is in the centers pertaining to the belly, the lower part of the body below the navel. This is of course where sexual energy and desires also live. We could even say that life force is the energy of sexuality, or more accurately that sexuality is an expression of life.

Desires are often the first step to creative consciousness because humans tend to do things they really want to do. The ability to act and have positive momentum is a yang quality that is ideally part of everyone's healthy daily existence.

For example, doing something that you really like—a hobby, a passion, a meaningful pursuit—can give you energy. Most parents know that if they tell their kids there will be ice cream or another favorite treat at the end of an activity, the kids are far more likely to be motivated and have energy for the task at hand.

Exerting effort to achieve something that you really want to do, a real project of passion, is often the best feeling there is, better than almost anything else.

Getting in touch with the feeling of wantings and desires in the belly does help to unlock vitality for some people. I know it did for me at key periods of my recovery and many others that I have worked with in IST sessions.

Connecting a person with the energy of wantings and desires can make a huge positive difference in their trajectory towards recovery, even if they are not yet ready to be physically active.

MANY TYPES OF DESIRES & WANTINGS, INCLUDING SOME THAT FALL FLAT OR OTHERS THAT PULL YOU AWAY

When I started to get sick with CFS, I felt as if I was living someone else's life but I didn't know it yet. At some point, though, after the years of striving to get my dream job, I realized the dream was empty. I lost any sense of purpose when I could no longer see my future in that career and still had no idea how to get out or where else I would be.

I recall sitting at the desk late in the evening working on a breaking news story, looking over at my editor and seeing the track I would take to becoming an editor of a financial newspaper. I knew that I did not want it. That track looked empty and lonely to me. I did not know what I wanted, but after that moment, I just could not go back to make myself want that track anymore.

It was not until I found meditation and IST that I would reclaim that drive again. And for me, when that bigger sense of purpose was not there, I had no direction; I had no reason to recover.

Now my life is so full, with a partner whom I adore, friends I love and cannot wait to share time with, a business that is all about helping people to shine in their own ways, and projects with numerous friends and contacts in the fields of meditation and personal transformation. Almost every day, I feel spontaneously full of joy and gratitude that often bubbles up in me when I am driving down the hill to my meditation class, with a view of the San Francisco Bay Area.

I never thought I would end up here, doing this, but I got here because I really let go of all the patterns and conditioning that said I should be that other person who got sick with CFS. I became more myself and figured out that this life is the one for me, and it is so energizing because it is filled with purpose, direction, and meaning.

This is a complicated thing to talk about because if you are super unwell with CFS, and it seems like you really want things, it makes no sense at all that wanting something more would make you better. In fact it could even be insulting to hear that getting in touch with a really deep wanting that can bring a sense of purpose or direction into your life could make you feel better.

The key is that this needs to be the kind of wanting that makes your life feel full of purpose and meaning, not an empty kind of desire that turns into dust when you get your hands onto it. When I say an empty desire, I mean something that you think you want, perhaps like a particular holiday, a new shiny gadget, or a better and bigger car when the one you have is fine. But when you get it, you realize that it is just something everyone else around you values, not necessarily wanting from deep inside of yourself.

FINDING DESIRES & WANTINGS THAT FILL YOU UP

Desire and wantings are interesting because when you really get into the felt sense of them in your body, they have energy. Some of our wantings and desires take us off track. You know the things that take us on a loop for days, weeks, or even years that we later regret and wonder why we did it.

When I had CFS, I remember getting into such a knot with myself wondering if I should go to a friend's birthday. Would I crash? Would it lift me up? Was it a terrible idea to go out and spend some time with some dear friends and laugh a bit?

It was a very difficult phase, as I would crash all the time and I was still subconsciously thinking somewhere inside that it was my fault. That I crashed because I had done something wrong. If only I could work out what I had done wrong, I could fix it and the crashing would stop. But more than that, I had no real strong sense of purpose in my life.

The thing is that at that time, I was so out of touch with what I really wanted. I felt lost and alone. And I did not know why I was so sick. Much of my strategy for getting better involved controlling the factors that I believed were making me sick. Food, alcohol, social time, even exercise and just going out to the mall. What I did not know at the time was that the urge to control all my choices, and limit myself to such a degree, was probably making me sicker.

When I moved towards the things that I really wanted from deep inside of myself, such as traveling to exotic places with beautiful landscapes and interesting people, I generally got better. Or when I started meditating on retreats, spending time in silence, just watching the breath and moving inside of myself, I got better. Even more than that, meditation allowed me to see a trajectory towards finding the things that helped me to get better, rather than being on a path of increasingly limiting everything that made me happy.

My experience of getting in touch with that energy of wantings and desires is that it is extremely invigorating.

I had so much fun in that initial phase of self-exploration, sourcing the blockages in my belly energy and releasing a lot of old stuff that I had been holding onto. Like so many modern people, I was holding onto an enormous amount of suppressed rage. I had twisted it in on myself and tied my belly centers in knots. Releasing it meant having session after session of going into the felt sense of the lower parts of my body and finding what was held in there. It was often accompanied by loud yelling, screaming, punching, hitting cushions and foam blocks.

I felt so alive, invigorated, and inspired when that suppressed intensity was released using the IST process.

The energy below the navel or the belly is like the engine for the body of life force. When it is suppressed and pushed down or tied in knots like mine was, there is a huge amount of vitality unavailable to us.

In contrast to the first few years, when I was really sick with CFS, I spent a lot of time going around in circles just not knowing what was right. Of course, the worrying did not prevent crashes; it probably made them worse. But like many people with CFS, I had this idea that if only I could control whatever it was that was causing the crash, then I would get better.

What I did not realize was that, in the control, I was pushing down the energy of wantings and desires and even my own willpower. This was suppressing the energy of life inside of me.

To get to that essence, there is a need to peel off the layers along the way. Sometimes this can be seen like peeling off layers of an onion to get to the essential core. The journey of spiritual transformation is one of getting to know and embrace all parts of ourselves. The good, the bad, the ugly. Including the thoughts and emotions, the life force, and also the timeless essence at the core.

FINDING PURPOSE

In my own journey, I had plenty of wanting and desire my whole life. I wanted to be a journalist and a writer, I wanted to travel the world, I wanted love. But it wasn't until I started to realize that I had an inner drive to meditate and practice inner transformation work that I really found a sense of meaning and purpose.

The meaning and purpose emerged in the middle of the phase of being really sick with CFS when I was in Malawi, Africa, my birthplace. I was sitting on the edge of Lake Malawi, feeling a sense of deep connection and inner silence that echoed through time. In that moment, I changed and became interested in finding this sense of connection everywhere in my life.

Later, when I had become passionate about IST and meditation and started to facilitate this work for clients and students, then I had a sense of a greater purpose outside of myself that brought more meaning than I could ever have imagined. In that sense of meaning and purpose, there was a direction, like a guiding light, that grounded me in myself and gave me energy.

Something that I found in common with many of the people who recovered from CFS/ME was that in the process of recovery, they discovered something that they really wanted and changed their lives to make it happen. In the process of that shift in orientating their lives towards getting what they really wanted, they recovered.

This step along the pathway of recovery has been one that I have contemplated a lot over the years. I saw it again and again with many case studies and clients, as well as in my own life. In that old saying, "actions speak louder than words," it is implied that will is needed to really see whether someone means what they say.

Will is the ability to get things done. Here I am using the word to talk about the force of willpower that is really a neutral aspect of our consciousness. It is not an emotion or a thought; it is a motion towards doing things. And it is a huge part of the human experience. Just look around at the world and all that people get done every day and every year and every decade. But when someone has CFS or burnout, the extreme level of fatigue means they cannot get simple things done in their lives. Recovery happens when they start to find pathways to engage this force again on a regular basis without having a backlash of symptoms in the following hours or days.

Through observing the results of many people's actions, and those who recovered from extreme levels of fatigue and crashing, I saw that will has an important part to play for so many on the healing journey. Therefore, I have included a number of stories of people who recovered by moving towards something that gave their lives real purpose and meaning.

CASE STUDY – ZACK FINDING HIS PURPOSE AND DRIVE

Take Zack for example, who was 19 years old when he first came to see me and very unwell with CFS. Zack was a young musician who had lost his father and grandfather the year before.

The death of his dad was a shock to everyone in the family including his two siblings and his mother. And Zack had also been very close to his grandfather who was a great supporter of his career as a guitarist and singer.

When his dad died, Zack's mom made a very difficult decision to sell the family home in Maine. She went on to buy a smaller duplex, creating a third devastating loss for Zack within eighteen months. He felt like the ground had been taken out from underneath him. At 17 years old, he was not ready to lose his dad, grandfather, and the beloved home where he grew up. In his own words, he was gutted and absolutely exhausted.

In the IST sessions, we had to go deep into Zack's experience of a ripping in his heart over the loss of his dad and grandpa , and even more with losing his childhood home. So often people judge their grief and sadness as being too big or unmanageable, and so they swallow it. This creates something that can feel like a heavy boulder in their gut or body of energy that has to be dragged around. Releasing that grief can be scary because it seems endless at the time. But when it is allowed to flow, it does gently release, and it will at one point be done. Especially if held in care and openness by someone who knows how to help the energy of those emotions flow out.

As Zack released his immense grief, he felt a sense of peace and connection mending his broken heart, and he began to see that there was something more to heal in his own energy as result of the losses.

Zack had been so deeply grounded in his home and was not ready to leave when his mom sold it. He was left with something of a gap in his lower centers of energy or the energy pertaining to his belly and below. We deduced together that there was a need to heal some of the centers below.

We spent quite a bit of time using the IST sessions diving into these centers of energy, helping Zack to take back his ownership of the power to ground and land into his life and his new home.

During this exploration, Zack's whole face would light up, and his energy become vibrant and energized whenever he started to talk about how much he really wanted to be a successful musician. He had been very talented when he was younger until he started to smoke weed in an attempt to drown his losses. As a result of smoking, he'd lost touch with his love of playing, performing, and creating music that had been so natural to him as a kid.

In the healing, his enthusiasm and aptitude for music began to return, and Zack saw that the talent he had was something to cultivate and nurture. It was not something that would always be there if he did not take care of his energy body. So he stopped smoking weed, enrolled in a college for music, and continued his work with IST and the Clairvision meditation techniques. And yes, his CFS did go away!

Once Zack achieved full recovery, he and his band made an album and began touring. As a result of the inner work that he had done, and the reclaiming of his vital energy through IST, Zack was able to create a life that was a real expression of his creative self.

CASE STUDY – ANGELA AND HER FAMILY

Angela recovered from CFS when she had her first child, even though she was unwell and wasn't sure if having a baby was really a good idea.

She was about 29 years old and a marketing executive in Sydney when I met her. She had come down with CFS after traveling to Asia and contracting an exotic tropical illness that was never fully diagnosed. It had been three years, and still she was not recovered. She did not really know why that was.

She slept terribly, or a lot. She was always exhausted, often had some kind of cold or flu symptoms, and was highly restricted in what she could eat. Prior to her trip to Indonesia three years earlier, she was healthy and living a full and active lifestyle.

When I met Angela in a café in Darlinghurst, Sydney, I could tell that she was a bright and bubbly person who was somewhat subdued from her experience with the illness. She had dialed her work schedule back to part-time and struggled even to get that done. But there was a light on her horizon. She had met someone, they were in love and getting married, and she wanted a baby.

Angela and I kept in touch for about a year after that, and next time that I met her, she had the baby and was fully recovered. She shone bright in our second meeting, clearly so happy with her new life. When I asked her what she thought had made her better, she said that she didn't really know, but somehow when she had her little boy, everything shifted for her.

"I had done a lot of different alternative therapies so it is possible that something worked or it was the accumulation of everything that I had done, but I do know that I was the happiest I have ever been in my life to have my little Jonathon. I am not saying happiness can cure you because this is a real illness, but something happened when I gave birth and my body changed. I did not have the CFS anymore."

Studies show that pregnancy can be pretty neutral in regard to impacting the symptoms for women with CFS.[82]

A study to be conducted by the Newcastle University and ME Association and announced on July 15, 2022 said that there has been very little investigation on the outcomes of pregnancy for women with CFS/ME.[83]

The few results so far of any investigation have been relatively neutral or mixed regarding whether or not pregnancy and birth can have a positive or negative impact on women with this illness.

The New Jersey Chronic Fatigue Association says that, *"ME/CFS symptoms tend to improve in about one-third of pregnant ME/CFS patients, are unchanged in about one-third and worsen in about one-third of them... Within weeks of delivery, at least half the mothers either relapse or feel worse than before the pregnancy."*[84]

---

82. Richard S. Schacterle and Anthony L. Komaroff, "A Comparison of Pregnancies That Occur Before and After the Onset of Chronic Fatigue Syndrome," Archives of Internal Medicine 164, no. 4 (February 23, 2004): 401, https://doi.org/10.1001/archinte.164.4.401.

83. "Announcement: The ME Association Funds New Study Examining Pregnancy in ME/CFS," The ME Association, July 20, 2022, https://meassociation.org.uk/2022/07/announcement-the-me-association-funds-new-study-examining-pregnancy-in-me-cfs.

84. Rosemary Underhill, "Pregnancy in Women with Chronic Fatigue Syndrome (ME/CFS)," accessed June 12, 2024, https://www.njcfsa.org/wp-content/uploads/2010/09/Pregnancy-in-Women-with-ME-CFS.pdf.

For Angela and a few other women that I worked with, getting pregnant and having the baby that they really wanted did make a huge positive difference in their symptoms, and for some it got rid of the CFS altogether. My observation was that for those women, having the baby was deeply motivating at an organic level of their willpower. Not only did they get what they wanted; they were able to connect with a new level of that force of wanting or desire to the point that it really created a major positive groove in their physical health. This does not happen for everyone, but it does happen for some women for sure.

CASE STUDY – LIVIA RECOVERING FROM CFS

Livia was 16 years old when she first came down with CFS. She was not diagnosed for many years because CFS was not a well-known diagnosis at that time. She recovered when she had her second baby at the age of 29 years old.

Livia told me that when she was pregnant with her first baby, she felt amazing, and her CFS symptoms had disappeared. However, the birth had been long and taxing so that when she had him, the illness also returned. At least until her second child arrived.

"When I had my second baby, I had a newborn and a toddler, and I still had more energy than I had ever had with CFS. I was super tired with the babies, but that is a different kind of fatigue. The brain fog with CFS is something different. It drains your life away. I never had that again after having my second boy."

Livia was a journalist and continued working through her first pregnancy teaching journalism and doing freelance work for the radio news programs. When she had her first child, she and her husband were living in Sydney in a small apartment. Within the first year, they moved out of the city to a small house in a coastal town six hours north. They quickly purchased a piece of land and started to build their own home from scratch. It was a straw-bale house, and Livia was doing a lot of the less heavy labor herself even while she was pregnant with her second child, and was looking after a small toddler. At six months of the pregnancy, she was putting mud on the walls of their new home, which required a not insignificant amount of labor.

When I was interviewing her, it was clear to me that this act of love, building her family home from scratch, was a pretty big act of will. The couple had very little money at that time, and they were getting building resources from scrap yards and even from the side of the road. Even so, they managed to build a beautiful house that looked something like a huge open church. It was no small task.

Livia chose to have that second baby at home. Her first baby had been born in a hospital after more than 36 hours of labor. It was exhausting and long, and in the end she needed an epidural to get through it. But still she wanted to have the second baby in her own house.

It struck me that this woman and her husband had an enormous amount of courage to do these things. Livia certainly surprised many people in her life.

By the time the second baby arrived, she had completed doula training, learning a lot about how to improve the birth experience and the pain, and she had a good midwife to help her during the labor. She had learned that fear makes the labor pains worse, and had techniques to choose another pathway than the fear.

She was also physically a lot stronger, simply from building her house with a small toddler at her side.

However, more than that, her determination to live this life with her husband and children was fierce. She had decided to live a life outside of the city, to work as a journalist, and to create a home with her partner.

The second birth was very quick. It took just six hours of labor for that baby to be born, and he came out without complications. She was able to have him in her new home, even though it was not fully completed. And that was the end of her CFS.

Livia did so much personal work on herself and physical labor towards creating the life that she really wanted. On top of that, she was highly motivated for the sheer love of her children. All of this ended up catapulting her into recovery from CFS in a way that was unexpected. She did not do any of these things just to recover. She did them because of how much she wanted those children and her family to work. She engaged a level of willpower that she had not previously even touched in her life, and she got better.

CASE STUDY- BELINDA FROM LAW TO POETRY

Belinda had worked very hard in her career. She was an in-house lawyer for a big corporation, but she hated it. She was also married to a man she loved and was desperate to have a baby with him. Unfortunately, the couple was unable to conceive, and even after a lot of treatments and trying numerous options via the medical system, they could not have a baby.

When I met her, Belinda was devastated about this. She had been through a dark depression and was suffering from overwhelming fatigue. Even while seeing a really great therapist, and undergoing treatment for her loss, she was still hardly able to get out of bed in the mornings.

Essentially, the thing that she wanted the most in the world was not going to happen. She wanted to have a baby. It was clear there was a lot of grief that needed to be released and healed. But her fatigue was more than that. Somehow when Belinda realized that she wasn't going to have the life she hoped for, she felt even more stuck in a job that was unsatisfying and just crashed.

Belinda explained to me that she had a big turnaround when she started to write poetry. It was a small thing, she said, but it meant the world to her. She loved reading and had always wanted to be a writer. She started to write poems on a daily basis, taking care to craft them with beauty, and she started to feel alive again, she said.

Her poems were exquisite, so much so that she started to win competitions and was published in a literary journal.

Within a year of diving into this important passion, Belinda quit her job as a lawyer and started to write full-time. She recovered from her crash and the huge amount of grief that she had processed in the two years that she was so ill. After another year or two, she and her husband were able to make the decision to adopt.

With Belinda's permission, I was able to talk with her therapist and ask about the recovery. Belinda's therapist told me that she felt Belinda had connected with something different inside of herself when she started to write poetry. "Prior to this, she was stuck in a life that was not a reflection of who she really was. Belinda has very sensitive, refined aspects of herself that appreciate beauty and subtlety in art, as well as other things. She is a tender person, with a lot of potential for deep levels of feeling, but her life did not have the scope for her to express that part of herself before she started to bring forward her creativity. Expressing the full spectrum of sensitivity through poetry gave Belinda a new lease on life. In her grief, she had felt something inside of her that no longer wanted to live if she could not have that baby. But the writing gave her a newfound hope, and so much more energy and joy. It was a delight to see her come back to herself through this process," the therapist said.

We have so many different aspects of ourselves inside that we sometimes get pulled into one or another part and ignore the rest. So someone can be a professional, a mother, a sports player or whatever it is, but then they are not living the full depths of their being. In the expression of the more unconscious aspects of ourselves through art or creativity, we get to be more.

Life can seem so limiting and shallow without the fullness of our whole being in expression. When we define our personality and our existence through one pathway of expression, perhaps our profession or our family roles, we are potentially living in a cage of sorts. All of us have so much more to contribute and become. For some people this is a burning passion, even if it is unconscious, so much so that they seem to shut down inside when unable to express it fully.

Many times I have seen people recover from CFS or other fatigue-related illnesses through awakening their creativity. Creativity can spark the life force just as sexuality can. Engaging in this spark of life and putting it into art, writing, music, or some kind of creative expression has led many people to recover fully.

When we think we cannot do something like creative expression, we are blocking a flow of energy within us.

11

THE POWER OF TRUTH

"There is no real protection but the power of Truth."[85]

Beyond the yinyang symbol and the aim for flow and positive engagement, there is a key for many in the quest for truth or integrity. What I mean here is that some people with CFS or burnout who are chronically crashing or collapsing find that they have fallen out of integrity with themselves, or lost track of their own inner knowing of truth in a fundamental way. When they reclaim this inner sense of wisdom and clarity, many people do find their way back to full health.

---

85. Samuel Sagan MD, *Awakening the Third Eye* (Roseville, N.S.W, Australia: Clairvision, 1997), 273.

Bill was 28 years old when he became very ill. He had been a world-class athlete for 10 years, and he thought of himself as being physically tough. He grew up in Los Angeles, in downtown Venice, and spent a lot of his youth either training or on the street, fighting.

One hot summer evening, he was on the boardwalk late at night and got into a fight with another guy who had pushed him, or looked at him the wrong way. He was so angry that night that the other tough guy was a great outlet. He beat the guy to a pulp, he told me, to the point that he knew he could have killed him.

The other guy ended up in hospital, but in the moment when Bill saw himself leaning over this man, looking into his cowering eyes and seeing the pain, terror and rage reflected his own, Bill knew he was done. He could not do this anymore; it was over. No more fights, he thought to himself in that moment. He knew in his gut and deep in his soul that this was wrong. Even though according to the street code that he had lived by since he was a kid, he was just being the king, making his own strength known and keeping himself and his buddies protected.

Three weeks later, Bill got sick, really really really sick. He came down with Lyme disease, mercury poisoning, and a bunch of other things, that made him mentally and physically ill. Some would have said that he had a breakdown. This super fit, superhuman guy who prided himself on his strength spent over 18 months in hell. His body broke down on him, his mind lurching into extreme neuroses such as paranoia and fear.

When we worked in IST a few years later, Bill saw that his decision to stop fighting had preceded his collapse. He had seen where his life was heading, and he knew that something inside of him had just flipped a switch and stopped the train that he was on.

The voice inside of him was not one that spoke in words; it was silent knowing. He just knew with a total certainty, even though listening to that voice seemed to cause him a whole lot of suffering, pain, and destruction. His whole life was built on fighting. Even the high-level sports that he had done for so many years came from that part of him that only knew how to fight and to win. Collapsing seemed to be the absolute worst thing that could have happened to him at the time. It was devastating.

Clairvision School has a saying to illustrate the power of that kind of inner knowing which can stop us in our tracks, "To see, is to know, is to be," illustrating that the power of being, seeing, and knowing are one. When you really see something, you know it. And that changes you. You become different. The ability to see like this is part of our very essence. Perhaps you could even say it is the part that is timeless and that exists beyond emotions and thoughts.

When I met Bill years later, he was on a completely different path. A path of healing and helping others around him to do the same. He was a coach, and had a tribe of his own followers who listened to his advice regarding their own journey of getting healthy. Through IST he had connected to the part of himself that valued truth and integrity more than winning, and then he went out there and lived this in his life, helping others to do the same.

In our IST session, Bill felt much relief and opening in his heart when he looked back at that younger self, seeing the turning point in his whole life trajectory. He was able to accept that he had made the decision to get off of the train of fighting and violence, and that it had taken a few years for the rest of him to catch up. Those years were spent first purging physically through the illnesses, the necessary changes in diet and lifestyle, and later cleansing his soul through deep emotional work. It was painful and scary, testing him in every way, but it had brought him closer to this inner knowing that we might call truth.

The inner knowing that told him to get off the train was a kind of clarity that everyone has, although many do not listen to it. It was something akin to sincerity, the part inside that really knows the truth no matter what other parts of the psyche have to say.

Sagan says:

For you see, you may not be a passionate lover of Truth, but your Higher Self is. Always. You may play games in your life, you may seek power for childish motivations, you may cover yourself in mud—in the background your

Higher Self will still be yearning for Truth and Truth alone. It does not matter where you as an individual may choose to go. Your Higher Self simply cannot move toward any other direction than Truth. That is Its imperishable nature.

Sagan points out that, *"If you are not after Truth, your Higher Self will start working against you... We would call this self-sabotage."*[86]

Bill was not concerned about being good or bad when he made that decision to stop the direction that he had been on since he was a kid. He was not making a moral decision. But from the most sincere part of himself, he silently just knew that it was a life built on falsehoods and did not feel right to continue.

I have met many people who felt that they learned a lot from the journey of recovering from CFS, myself included. It can be delicate to discuss this because few people (if anyone) would consciously make themselves that sick on purpose, even if it was in order to find their truth. I am not suggesting this at all. But it seems to be part of the human experience to learn and grow through difficult times, and when people are able to do this, they are typically thankful for what they have gained.

---

86. Samuel Sagan MD, *Awakening the Third Eye* (Roseville, N.S.W, Australia: Clairvision, 1997), 273.

For myself and Bill, and maybe even you too, the journey of recovery was one that opened up possibilities of connection to the most sincere aspects of the inner self.

It turned out that for me, I did not want a good life. I wanted a life that allowed me to be me, that felt good from the inside, from that part of me that has clarity and knows a higher sense of spiritual Truth.

The journey of recognizing one's own inner truth and a step towards a higher standpoint of real spiritual Truth with a capital T is a long and in my view very beautiful and rewarding path. Yet it starts here and now, right where you are, reading this book today.

For me finding that connection to the inner knowing that was pulling me in a different direction was not an easy journey. And it did involve recovering from CFS, but it was also about learning to value that sense of my own sense of inner truth, even when it went against common sense.

Mother, a spiritual teacher formerly known as Mirra Alfassa who joined Sri Aurobindo in India to run his ashram until she left her body Nov. 17, 1973, said in May 1954, *"The truth is in us; we have only to become aware of it."*[87]

Sagan says, *"Actually, before you can grasp Truth with a capital T, you have to start with being true to yourself."* He describes this quality of being true to yourself as more

---

87. "Truth and Speech," Words of the Mother - Truth and Speech, accessed June 11, 2024, https://library.sriaurobindoashram.org/mother/cwm14/chapter/36/.

recognizable by the term sincerity: *"Sincerity is of another nature. Deep inside some things feel right, and some other things feel wrong... It doesn't scream inside like certain desires. You have to listen to it carefully."*[88]

CASE STUDY – BILL FOLLOWING TRUTH AND COMING TO TERMS WITH HIS OWN VIOLENCE

Bill's journey of awakening and healing included learning to identify and listen to this voice. At first, we had many IST sessions where Bill had heard the knowing inside of himself that something was not right but he did it anyway, and got sick as a result.

During that phase, he was often also paranoid that this or that thing he was doing might be right or wrong, good or bad. But he became more confident in hearing the sincerity inside of himself, learning that it was not something that came with a charge of fear or other emotions. It was quiet and simple.

One example was walking into a building where there were numerous perverse presences, knowing that it was not a good place to sleep, but doing it anyway because he wanted to make his girlfriend happy. The result was getting ill for a few weeks.

---

88. Samuel Sagan MD, *Awakening the Third Eye* (Roseville, N.S.W, Australia: Clairvision, 1997), 275.

In these cases when he made a mistake and listened to his desires and fears rather than the simplicity of the sincere inner knowing, there was no need for punishment. Often, he would feel that he should punish himself or others for the mistake. But no, the best thing to do was to see what happened and then take it as a learning to listen next time.

Over time, Bill learned to listen to that sincerity inside of himself and make decisions from there. Sometimes this meant that he did not know the answer immediately; he had to give himself time to find the clarity. Other times, he needed to call me for a session or speak to a good friend who could reflect him because he knew that emotions were in the way of his ability to hear his own wisdom.

Bill learned that the true power inside of himself was his vulnerability. On the streets he had learned to cover that up at all costs, to put it aside and exhibit only strength to those around him to the point that he had almost completely closed to the vulnerability.

Getting so sick for those years and seeing his life shatter in front of him put Bill on his knees, and also brought him to a place where he could be vulnerable and even see the real strength in that level of vulnerability.

Vulnerability is something that we are told is a weakness. It makes us prey to others, we are told by the world and the dictionary. However, when we can turn with real self-awareness towards our own wounds, and allow the depths of feeling there to be seen and felt, we can also know our own essence and connect with this sincerity that keeps us safe and on the right track. In fact, it takes courage to let yourself be vulnerable.

In my experience, awareness is not static; it grows and expands as you apply it in your life and in yourself. A bit like a muscle that you build over time. Except that it perhaps has no limits, where a muscle can only really get so strong even after a lot of time and a lot of practice.

Tenzin Palmo, a Buddhist nun who was born in England whose calling to become a Tibetan Buddhist led her to meditate for 12 years in a cave in the snow, talks about the emergence of silent knowing as you move into awareness in meditation.

She points out that silent knowing is our birthright, yet as human beings we spend so much of our time outside of this vast sense of inner wisdom that is innate to our awareness, carried away by emotions, thoughts, and the distractions of our environment.

> *Behind the constant flow of our thoughts and our feelings and our emotions, there is that quality of knowing that we usually don't recognize because we are so caught up in the thinking. And we don't recognize that which is behind the thoughts which in a way is the quality emanating the thoughts, that quality of clarity and empty spaciousness behind the coming and going of the thoughts. And in the Tibetan tradition, this is compared to being the sky.*

Because especially in Tibet, the skies are vast and endless. The sky has no circumference; it is infinite. You can't divide it up and say that's my bit of space, that's your bit of space. It's something which we all share together. And so this is therefore a very good simile of the nature of the mind which has no center and has no ending. But of course the mind is not exactly like space because the mind has awareness. It has the clarity, that sense of cognitive knowing. But that sense of unborn awareness, which in Mahayana Buddhism is called the Buddha nature, is that which unites us with all existence, not just human beings but everything, because as I say, it has no boundaries so in that state of primordial awareness, there is no I and other. Essentially, duality doesn't exist. There is just the quality of knowing of being very aware and very open and spacious mind. So in that sense you could call that a state of one-ness.[89]

For me the journey to recovering from CFS was very much one of learning to come back and back again and again to this sense of silent inner knowing and clarity. From that standpoint, I learned to see what was happening in the collapsing and could choose something else.

---

89. Tenzin Palmo, "The Nature of the Mind," Global Oneness Project, uploaded June 22, 2007, https://www.youtube.com/watch?v=sOsQa7sf6FE.

Often after I had crashed, I would realize I had somehow missed something important that I had needed or not done, which had then somehow contributed to the onset of the collapsing mechanism. Talking about this is slippery ground as it is so easy to get into some moral judgment of what is right and wrong, even going down the track of punishing myself for not doing something correctly.

I had to learn the difference between really seeing and knowing from that standpoint of neutral clarity and the psychology of self-punishment and doubt that always ended up in unnecessary suffering.

In the Clairvision style of work, the centers of energy above the head are referred to as verticality. This can be seen as a metaphor, just as the sky is a metaphor for spacious awareness. But it works in a very experiential way, because when you put your awareness above, it is really easy to just feel yourself as vertical or not vertical.

In the verticality above, there is a simple sense of the same inner knowing and clarity that Tenzin Palmo talks about, the sincerity of that wisdom that is above. There are some people, myself included, for whom falling out of alignment with that straightness of the objective sense of inner wisdom can create a collapse.

Bill, for example, was so offtrack from that inner knowing or wisdom that he nearly killed a man. As he was beating that guy from the suburbs on that hot summer night, he knew that he could kill him right there and then. That was a shocking moment for Bill to such a degree that his ordinary thoughts dropped away, and the clouds parted in his consciousness. The light of inner wisdom shined through. He could see just for that moment how offtrack he really was.

Could we say that the next few years of illness, suffering, and pain were caused by that brilliant light of clarity that shone through him in that one moment? I could not say that. Rather, it was because he had shut down the intense force of the violence that was so alive and unbridled when he was a fighter. That intense force had stayed inside, creating an inner pressure that continually ate away at him, and contributed to an intense illness that lasted until he learned to hold it differently inside of himself. Bill used the IST sessions to learn how to stay connected to his own sense of truth and open to that intense force inside of himself, grounding in his own density instead of just reacting from the violence for the sake of it.

But Bill himself saw a correlation with his path of understanding integrity through his own experience and his recovery when he was in IST sessions with me. And it is not to say that he felt grateful for all the pain that had ensued, because he was truly beaten by that phase of illness and extreme neurosis. But he was somewhere glad that he had been led to a path where he could make his own inner knowing and connection to Truth central to his whole life without shutting down his immense intensity that was previously expressed through fighting.

CASE STUDY – RICHARD'S SPIRITUAL CONNECTION AND RECOVERY FROM CFS

For Richard, spiritual awakening was also an important part of recovery. His crystallization was really an intense grasping that caused a lot of pain and at times extreme tension in his body. When we used IST to source the extreme tendency to grip his whole body like a fist held constantly tight, it became clear that he was also cutting off at a very deep level from anything spiritual, or even the most mundane levels of love.

Richard was very open about the fact that he did not really feel anything apart from this grasping and tension in his body. He had difficulty with any emotion other than frustration. He was pretty much emotionally numb. He had a girlfriend for whom he was extremely grateful, and experienced care, but he could not share in her love, he told me.

In this system of subtle bodies, the whole body of energy and the emotions and thoughts work together with the physical. They are not completely separate. It is a holistic approach to the human being.

In addition to all of those parts, there is another aspect that this system calls the higher ego, the spiritual part of the human. Experientially, this often becomes tangible when there is a moment of complete silence, and the thoughts do not chatter on. In the silence there is fullness, and even a sense of Peace. It is a moment when we feel ourselves as vast or full of love or wonder, something that many of us really long for.

Richard responded to the silence and peace in the IST sessions when we created a meditative space of connection, but as soon as he came out, he would start grasping. Using the regression technique, we found that there was a past life long ago when Richard had made a very strong decision to never turn towards the light again. In that life he had watched some people torture and kill his wife, and although they left him to live, he was dead inside. He had made a very clear decision to cut off from the light inside of himself because he felt so deeply betrayed and let down by what he thought was God.

This betrayal continued to play out in his current life through his sense of total bitterness about authorities, about his schooling, about his parents. He had strong conspiracy theories that he adhered to through almost every decision he made. It was extremely painful, but he was convinced it was true.

As we worked through the past life events again and again, Richard began to feel himself as more than this intense level of grasping and bitterness. He started to feel where he had been connected to the light. Things began to open up and soften in his psyche, and he was able to continue to build his subtle bodies through the uplifting and regain his strength completely.

In my own journey, looking back at that young woman who was thrashing about doing financial journalism, motivated largely by external drivers for success and recognition, yet so desolate with the emptiness of all of that, I am glad that I have been taken on such a different journey. A journey that neither I nor my family nor any of my childhood friends could have ever imagined.

I cannot separate out the experience of learning to grow in the awareness of my own truth inside of myself from the meditation practices that I have learned with the Clairvision style of work, which strengthened and fortified my subtle bodies. The cultivation of subtle bodies and continual alignment with Truth at the level of the sky go together for me and in this style of practice.

I was able to step into more and more intensity in my life without crashing as I learned to retain conscious awareness in this state of clarity for longer and longer periods of time. My awareness muscle, if you like, became more available and steady.

In many ways it is pretty similar to physical exercise, where I also had to build my strength incrementally, bit by bit until I had more physical stamina after CFS. Even though I had been very athletic and active prior to having CFS, my physical abilities were almost totally lost. Building that back up took sustained effort and patience.

ADDENDUM – WITH A LITTLE HELP FROM MY FRIENDS

Most importantly, recovery through seeing and addressing these deep patterns internally requires patience, and everyone benefits from having the right support. Friends that help you to see your true self, and support your journey are a key aspect of making these shifts in a sustainable and ongoing way.

Please remember while you are on your pathway to recovery that building the capacity for awareness and cultivating your life force energy does take time and a lot of help from the kind of friends and colleagues who love you and want you to really shine your true self in your life.

As one of my favorite artists, Bill Withers says in his song 'Lean on Me' released in April 1972, "We all need somebody to lean on." In my experience we need more than one person who can hold your highest self in mind, and encourage you to keep going forward in your recovery journey even when you fall down.

The CDC says that although it is hard to measure the effects of isolation and loneliness, studies do show that these conditions put people's health and wellbeing at serious risk.[90]

---

90. "Loneliness and Social Isolation Linked to Serious Health Conditions," Centers for Disease Control and Prevention, April 29, 2021, https://www.cdc.gov/aging/publications/features/lonely-older-adults.html.

The CDC points to this issue impacting older folks, but in truth this is a condition that brings down anyone at any age.[91] According to a study in the *Interactive Journal of Medical Research*,

> *Loneliness is a global health epidemic that affects a significant number of global populations. In the United States, an estimated 17% of adults aged 18 to 70 years report loneliness. Monetary loss as a result of loneliness is estimated to be between US$8074.80 and US$12,0777.70 per person per year in the United Kingdom. The monetary cost of lost days and loss in productivity is estimated to be US$3.14 billion per year for employees in the United Kingdom. Loneliness is also linked to a 30% increase in heart disease, stroke, dementia, depression, and anxiety.*[92]

While loneliness is not necessarily a cause of CFS, ME or burnout, addressing isolation or any stubborn idea that you have to go it on your own, will help your healing journey immeasurably. I wholeheartedly recommend that you put time and effort into creating a community of people around you who uplift your spirits and bring you hope.

---

91. Amy Novotny, "The Risks of Social Isolation," Monitor on Psychology, May 2019, https://www.apa.org/monitor/2019/05/ce-corner-isolation.

92. Hurmat Ali Shah and Mowafa Househ, "Understanding Loneliness in Younger People: Review of the Opportunities and Challenges for Loneliness Interventions," *Interactive Journal of Medical Research*, 12 (November 2, 2023), https://doi.org/10.2196/45197.

A GLIMPSE OF WHAT COMES NEXT: FREE RESOURCES

Thank you for buying this book, *Reclaiming Vitality: A Healing Journey Through Chronic Fatigue and Burnout.*

I have a gift that will help you in your journey, a free video about technology and managing your energy online:

www.samanthakeen.com/book_gift

BIBLIOGRAPHY

"About Us." Center for Humane Technology. Accessed July 8, 2024. https://www.humanetech.com/who-we-are.

Agle, Raelan. *Finding Freedom: Escaping From the Prison of Chronic Fatigue Syndrome.* Editor Dr. D. Olson Pook. (N.P. Dec 2019)

"Announcement: The ME Association Funds New Study Examining Pregnancy in ME/CFS." The ME Association, July 20, 2022. https://meassociation.org.uk/2022/07/announcement-the-me-association-funds-new-study-examining-pregnancy-in-me-cfs.

Barsam, Tayebeh, Mohammad Reza Monazzam, Ali Akbar Haghdoost, Mohammad Reza Ghotbi, and Somayeh Farhang Dehghan. "Effect of Extremely Low Frequency Electromagnetic Field Exposure on Sleep Quality in High Voltage Substations." Iranian Journal of Environmental Health Science & Engineering, November 30, 2012. https://www.ncbi.nlm.nih.gov/pmc/articles/pmc3561068/.

"Buddha's Enlightenment." Kadampa Buddhism, March 13, 2023. https://kadampa.org/reference/buddhas-enlightenment).

"Burn-out an 'Occupational Phenomenon': International Classification of Diseases." World Health Organization, May 28, 2019. https://www.who.int/news/item/28-05-2019-burn-out-an-occupational-phenomenon-international-classification-of-diseases.

"Chaos Definition & Meaning." Merriam-Webster. Accessed June 11, 2024. https://www.merriam-webster.com/dictionary/chaos.

"Chinese Traditional Medicine." U.S. National Library of Medicine. Accessed June 11, 2024. https://www.nlm.nih.gov/exhibition/chinesemedicine/yin_yang.html.

Dean, Brian. "Zoom User Stats: How Many People Use Zoom?" Backlinko, February 13, 2024. https://backlinko.com/zoom-users.

Evers, Stefan, Marthe Fischera, Arne May, and Klaus Berger. "Prevalence of Cluster Headache in Germany: Results of the Epidemiological DMKG Study." Journal of Neurology, Neurosurgery, and Psychiatry, November 2007. https://www.ncbi.nlm.nih.gov/pmc/articles/PMC2117619.

"Fast Facts: ME/CFS." Centers for Disease Control and Prevention, May 30, 2024. https://www.cdc.gov/me-cfs/about/fast-facts-about-me-cfs.html.

Freudenberger, Herbert J. "Staff Burn-out." *Journal of Social Issues* 30, no. 1 (January 1974): 159–65. https://doi.org/10.1111/j.1540-4560.1974.tb00706.x.

Hao, Karen. "The Facebook Whistleblower Says Its Algorithms Are Dangerous. Here's Why." MIT Technology Review, June 29, 2022. https://www.technologyreview.com/2021/10/05/1036519/facebook-whistleblower-frances-haugen-algorithms/.

Harvey, S. B., M. Wadsworth, S. Wessely, and M. Hotopf. "The Relationship between Prior Psychiatric Disorder and Chronic Fatigue: Evidence from a National Birth Cohort Study." *Psychological Medicine* 38, no. 7 (November 2, 2007): 933–40. https://doi.org/10.1017/s0033291707001900.

Hughes, Bettany. *Venus and Aphrodite: A Biography of Desire.* New York: Basic Books, 2020.

"Is Staying up Late Similar to Being Drunk?" Creyos, April 25, 2024. https://creyos.com/resources/articles/staying-up-late-same-as-being-drunk.

Lee, Jena. "A Neuropsychological Exploration of Zoom Fatigue." Psychiatric Times, November 17, 2020. https://www.psychiatrictimes.com/view/psychological-exploration-zoom-fatigue.

Leswing, Kif. "Why We're Experiencing 'Zoom Fatigue' and How to Fix It." CNBC, February 25, 2021. https://www.cnbc.com/2021/02/25/zoom-fatigue-why-we-have-it-how-to-fix-it.html.

Leunig, Michael. "Prayers." Leunig. Accessed June 11, 2024. https://www.leunig.com.au/works/prayers.

Levine, Peter A., and Chris Sorensen. *Waking the Tiger: Healing Trauma*. Solon, OH: Findaway World, LLC, 2017.

Li, Choh-Luh. "A Brief Outline of Chinese Medical History with Particular Reference to Acupuncture." *Perspectives in Biology and Medicine* 18, no. 1 (September 1974): 132–43. https://doi.org/10.1353/pbm.1974.0013.

Lindner, Jannik. "Must-Know Burnout Statistics [Recent Analysis]." GITNUX, May 27, 2024. https://blog.gitnux.com/burnout-statistics/.

"Loneliness and Social Isolation Linked to Serious Health Conditions." Centers for Disease Control and Prevention, April 29, 2021. https://www.cdc.gov/aging/publications/features/lonely-older-adults.html.

Lusk, Jayson. "The Evolution of American Agriculture." Jayson Lusk, June 27, 2016. http://jaysonlusk.com/blog/2016/6/26/the-evolution-of-american-agriculture.

Martin, Douglas. "Herbert Freudenberger, 73, Coiner of 'Burnout,' Is Dead." *New York Times*, December 5, 1999, sec. 1.

"ME/CFS Basics." Centers for Disease Control and Prevention, May 10, 2024. https://www.cdc.gov/me-cfs/about/index.html.

Miller, Lisa. *The Awakened Brain: The New Science of Spirituality and Our Quest for an Inspired Life*. New York: Random House, 2021.

Miller, Lisa, and Teresa Barker. *The Spiritual Child: The New Science on Parenting for Health and Lifelong Thriving*. New York: Picador/St. Martin's Press, 2016.

"A Netflix Original Documentary." The Social Dilemma, March 14, 2022. https://www.thesocialdilemma.com/.

"Noble Definition & Meaning." Merriam-Webster. Accessed June 11, 2024. https://www.merriam-webster.com/dictionary/noble.

Novotny, Amy. "The Risks of Social Isolation." Monitor on Psychology, May 2019. https://www.apa.org/monitor/2019/05/ce-corner-isolation.

"Nyx." *Encyclopædia Britannica*, May 20, 2024. https://www.britannica.com/topic/Nyx.

Palmo, Tenzin. "The Nature of the Mind." Global Oneness Project. Uploaded June 22, 2007. YouTube video, https://www.youtube.com/watch?v=sOsQa7sf6FE.

Paul, Kari. "'It Let White Supremacists Organize': The Toxic Legacy of Facebook's Groups." *The Guardian*, February 4, 2021. https://www.theguardian.com/technology/2021/feb/04/facebook-groups-misinformation.

Petersen, Anne Helen. *Can't Even: How Millennials Became the Burnout Generation*. London: Vintage Digital, 2021.

Robinson, Bryan. "New Outlook on Burnout for 2023: Limitations on What Managers Can Do." *Forbes*, September 12, 2023. https://www.forbes.com/sites/bryanrobinson/2023/02/07/new-outlook-on-burnout-for-2023-limitations-on-what-managers-can-do/?sh=6cc56d724343.

Sagan, Samuel, MD. *A Language to Map Consciousness.* Point Horizon Institute. 1996 - 2023. Accessed June 11, 2024. https://clairvision.org/books/altmc/a-language-to-map-consciousness.html.

Sagan, Samuel, MD. *Awakening the Third Eye.* Roseville, N.S.W, Australia: Clairvision, 1997.

Sagan, Samuel, MD. *Entity Possession: Freeing the Energy Body of Negative Influences.* Rochester, Vt: Destiny Books, 1997.

Sagan, Samuel, MD. *KT Flow of Life.* Point Horizon Institute, 2011. Written PDF for audio recordings on an online correspondence course.

Sagan, Samuel, MD. *KT FuXi's Mountain.* Point Horizon Institute. 2011. Written PDF for the audio online correspondence course.

Sagan, Samuel, MD. *KT Subtle Bodies, the Fourfold Model.* Point Horizon Institute. 2011. Written PDF for the audio recorded online correspondence course.

Sagan, Samuel. *Regression: Past-life Therapy for Here and Now Freedom.* Roseville, N.S.W: Clairvision, 1996.

Satprem. *Sri Aurobindo, or, the Adventure of Consciousness.* Delhi, Mysore: Mother's Institute of Research and Mira Aditi, 2008.

Schacterle, Richard S., and Anthony L. Komaroff. "A Comparison of Pregnancies That Occur before and after the Onset of Chronic Fatigue Syndrome." *Archives of Internal Medicine* 164, no. 4 (February 23, 2004): 401. https://doi.org/10.1001/archinte.164.4.401.

Shah, Hurmat Ali, and Mowafa Househ. "Understanding Loneliness in Younger People: Review of the Opportunities and Challenges for Loneliness Interventions." *Interactive Journal of Medical Research* 12 (November 2, 2023). https://doi.org/10.2196/45197.

Shakya, Holly B., and Nicholas A. Christakis. "Association of Facebook Use with Compromised Well-Being: A Longitudinal Study." *American Journal of Epidemiology* 185, no. 3 (January 16, 2017): 203–11. https://doi.org/10.1093/aje/kww189.

Shan, Jun. "What Do Yin and Yang Represent?" ThoughtCo, June 7, 2024. https://www.thoughtco.com/yin-and-yang-629214.

Singer, Michael A. *The Untethered Soul: The Journey beyond Yourself*. Oakland, CA: Noetic

Books, Institute of Noetic Sciences, New Harbinger Publications, Inc, 2013.

Smith, Kate. "Women Experience Higher Levels of 'Zoom Fatigue' than Men, Study Finds." CBS News, April 21, 2021. https://www.cbsnews.com/news/zoom-fatigue-women-higher-men/.

Smith, Lisa. "Everything You Wanted to Know about Sex and Migraines (but Were Afraid to Ask!)." Association of Migraine Disorders, February 23, 2024. https://www.migrainedisorders.org/everything-you-wanted-to-know-about-sex-and-migraines-but-were-afraid-to-ask/.

Stockton, Nick. "What's up with That: Why Does Sleeping in Just Make Me More Tired?" Wired, July 22, 2014. https://www.wired.com/2014/07/whats-up-with-that-why-does-sleeping-in-just-make-me-more-tired/.

Suleyman, Mustafa, and Michael Bhaskar. *The Coming Wave: AI, Power and the Twenty-First Century's Greatest Dilemma.* London: Jonathan Cape, 2023.

"Truth and Speech." Words of the Mother - Truth and Speech. Accessed June 11, 2024. https://library.sriaurobindoashram.org/mother/cwm14/chapter/36/.

Underhill, Rosemary. "Pregnancy in Women with Chronic Fatigue Syndrome (ME/CFS)." Accessed June 12, 2024. https://www.njcfsa.org/wp-content/uploads/2010/09/Pregnancy-in-Women-with-ME-CFS.pdf.

Walker, Matthew P. *Why We Sleep: Unlocking the Power of Sleep and Dreams.* New York, NY: Scribner, an imprint of Simon & Schuster, Inc, 2018.

Walker, Matthew. "Matthew Walker's Defense of Napping: 5 Benefits of Napping - 2024." MasterClass, June 7, 2021. https://www.masterclass.com/articles/matthew-walkers-defense-of-napping.

Wang, Robin. *Yinyang: The Way of Heaven and Earth in Chinese Thought and Culture.* Cambridge: Cambridge University Press, 2012.

Wilhelm, Richard, trans. *I Ching or the Book of Changes.* Arkana, 1989.

ACKNOWLEDGEMENTS

It is hard to describe how it feels to complete a project that started over 20 years ago. Put simply, I feel an enormous amount of gratitude for all the help and the learning that happened to get me here, even if it took a lot longer than I, or anyone else around me, thought it would.

Most of all, my heart is full of love for my teacher, Dr. Samuel Sagan, who, though he passed away in 2016, directly mentored and helped me on this project in the early years of my work. Samuel's giving to me and so many others is impossible to measure.

Also to dear Ruth-Helen Camden, IST practitioner and psychologist, who really ignited my recovery and supported my entry into a spiritual life wholeheartedly. Finally, but not only because there are many more, I want to express my thanks to Brian Dooley who is an editor extraordinaire and a great human, without whom the last phases of this project would not have happened.

Many other people have supported me, mentored me and been wonderful clients along the way. In receiving all of that help and support, I was also deeply transformed and changed. It takes a village, and in my opinion that village is full of the power of love.

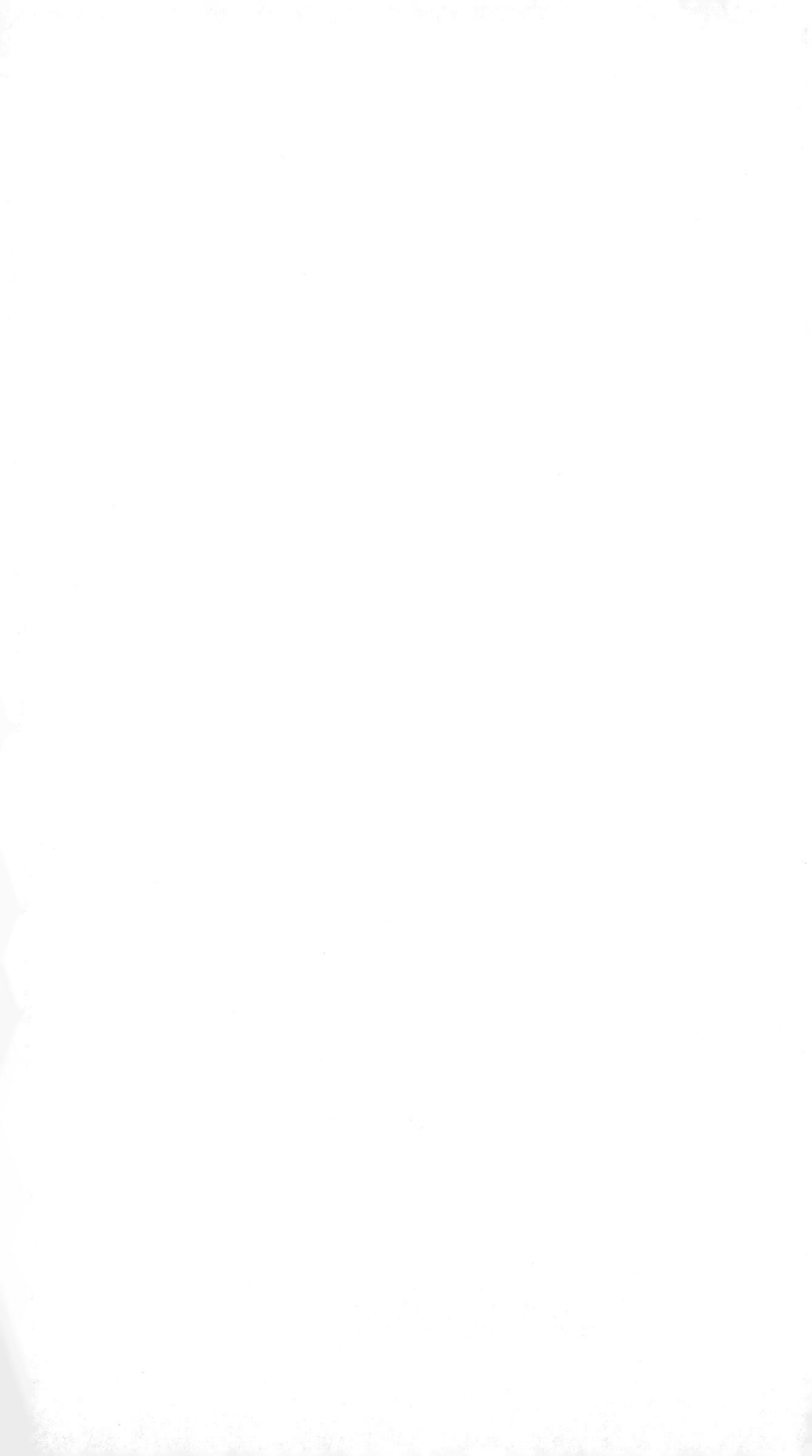

Made in the USA
Middletown, DE
25 October 2024